Basic
Orthopedic
Exams

Basic Orthopedic Exams

Zachary Child, M.D.

Resident in Orthopedic Surgery
University of New Mexico

Wolters Kluwer | Lippincott Williams & Wilkins
Health

Philadelphia · Baltimore · New York · London
Buenos Aires · Hong Kong · Sydney · Tokyo

Acquisitions Editor: Donna Balado
Managing Editor: Kelly Horvath
Marketing Manager: Jennifer Kuklinski
Production Editor: Gina Aeillo
Designer: Theresa Mallon
Compositor: Circle Graphics
Printer: R.R. Donnelley & Sons–Crawfordsville

Library of Congress Cataloging-in-Publication Data

Child, Zachary.
  Basic orthopedic exams / Zachary Child.
      p. ; cm.
  Includes index.
  ISBN-13: 978-0-7817-6333-2
  ISBN-10: 0-7817-6333-9
  1.   Orthopedics--Diagnosis. 2.   Physical diagnosis.   I. Title.
  [DNLM: 1.   Bone Diseases—diagnosis. 2.   Joint Diseases—diagnosis. 3.
Orthopedic Procedures—methods. 4.   Physical Examination—methods.   WE
225 C536b 2008]
  RD734.C45 2008
  616.7'075—dc22

                                                                    2006100664

07 08 09 10
1 2 3 4 5 6 7 8 9 10

Preface

This pocket book is not intended to be a definitive reference or source of orthopaedic examinations. Rather, it is an outgrowth of my own personal need to have a concise reference *with pictures* of a solid, basic orthopaedic examination; key items of a radiologic diagnosis; and whatever else has been important to me while rotating through and working in orthopaedics. The text is not exceptionally original, although the pictures are my own. The material is intended to address the particular needs of the upper-level medical student and non-orthopaedist (e.g., emergency medicine physician or family practitioner) and is put into my own words and understanding. My own experience witnessing a frustrated orthopaedist taking a verbal report of a consultation from a clinician not well versed in the language of orthopaedics was another source of inspiration for this book.

I make no claims to being an expert in this material. This material is based on notes from many sources and the expertise of practicing orthopaedists. Begun during my third year of medical school, this project was carried up until the beginning of my orthopaedic residency. The general goal of the book is to provide an outline of a concise orthopaedic examination according to body part with illustrations. It is accompanied by anatomic correlations for visual learners (like myself), and it provides basic information regarding common problems. The chapters all follow a basic pattern, starting with anatomy, which I think is the highest yield subject in orthopaedics. The material is not meant as a complete anatomic reference but, rather, as a brief review of relevant clinical anatomy. This is followed by a bulleted list of examination procedures for quick reference, followed in turn by text providing illustration and more details. Then, key radiologic findings for that section are provided, along with basic methods for interpreting plain-film radiographs. Finally, each chapter includes common orthopaedic fractures and dislocation patterns as well as musculoskeletal disease states.

For me, the artwork is a labor of love and is purposefully neoclassical. I am myself a one-time aspiring artist who has combined this with my love of anatomy and classical medical illustration to produce these figures. They are purposeful imitations of the style of da Vinci, Reubens, Michelangelo, Titian, and other great masters. If you are familiar with these artists, you may notice a blatant rip-off here and there. I ask for indulgence in this style from you, the reader, to convey accurate information in a way that I find aesthetically pleasing.

Hope this helps,

Zack

Acknowledgments

I would very much like to thank Drs. Dean Stites, Anthony Zissimos, and Ted Lange. Dr. Eberhardt Sauerland (*Grant's Atlas of Anatomy*, Dissector) also was an inspiring anatomist and teacher. I owe a great deal to Dr. Robert Schenck and Dr. Robert Quinn in New Mexico for giving me the opportunity to follow my dreams in orthopaedics as a surgeon and fellow artist. Finally, there is not enough room to thank my parents and my son for all their love and support.

Contents

6   Wrist and Hand   140

7   Hip   177

8   Knee   203

9 Foot and Ankle 232

1

Basic Approach

ANATOMY

Actually, not much is contained in this introductory chapter that is not adequately covered by a standard physical examination text; however, some information deserves repeating for emphasis. In orthopaedics, the basic approach to the patient begins with a solid appreciation of anatomy. This knowledge helps translate the patient's complaints into an appreciation of the structures that pertain to the location of that complaint. A good understanding of the neuroanatomic network that feeds muscular and cutaneous distributions aids a great deal in localizing a problem. **For medical students who are interested in orthopaedics and are preparing for rotations or electives, reviewing anatomy is by far the single best use of their time.** At later stages, a good education in anatomy is the foundation of an astute surgeon who is mindful of what areas to explore—and to avoid! A mentor once said that at heart, "all orthopaedists share a love of anatomy," which is certainly true for a great many surgeons. For the specialist or generalist who deals with orthopaedic complaints but does not treat them surgically, speaking the language of anatomy helps in communicating with the orthopaedist and guides the caregiver toward the correct diagnosis.

The high-yield areas of orthopaedic anatomy help localize problems and are relatively accessible topics. The dermatomal charts, which are familiar to every medical student but, perhaps, are not committed to memory, should be memorized. If the lesion is associated with the spine or spinal pathology needs to be ruled out, then dermatomes are essential. Spinal reflexes also correspond to specific locations and can help focus a complaint.

The course of major peripheral nerves also is essential. Orthopaedic emergencies often center around the identification of nerve-threatening injuries that could lead to long-term disability. The myotomal distribution of the great nerves of the body—the sciatic, sural, radial, ulnar, median, axillary, and musculocutaneous—are essential items of knowledge and focus in the examination. Knowledge

1

of vascular anatomy is helpful in the operating room and is the focus of countless "PIMP" questions for the student. Each chapter in this book will begin with a review of basic anatomy and pertinent structures.

PHYSICAL EXAMINATION

Patient History

As axiomatic as it may sound, the value of a good patient history cannot be overstated. The chief complaint and pertinent history guide the physical examination, invoke the mechanism of injury, and give a sense of urgency to the job at hand. The history often begs the diagnosis, and the mechanism of injury should fit the complaint and the examination findings. A good history and physical examination usually are very sensitive and specific for picking up the correct diagnosis in orthopaedics. All pain should have some version of the PQRST mnemonic recorded (Table 1.1).

Inspection

In most settings, whether the office, the wards, or the emergency department, removal of clothing can be easily accomplished and can add a great deal to your examination. The initial inspection looks for:

- **Obvious deformities:** Many patients arrive in the emergency department with something obviously "not right." A complete examination is still necessary, however, because some insults are part of an injury pattern, which entails additional injuries.
- **Swelling:** If possible, distinguish between focal and diffuse swelling. Whether swelling is proximal to a joint or intra-articular is extremely important. If so, is it warm to the touch, implying

Table 1.1 Pain Scale Using the PQRST Mnemonic

P	Pain (location)
Q	Quality (sharp, dull ache, locking, popping)
R	Radiation (is this referred pain? pain that is not musculoskeletal)
S	Severity (on a scale of 1–10, with 10 being the worst pain imaginable)
T	Time (how long since onset, duration, waxing/waning versus constant)

inflammation or infection? Is joint function or range of motion (ROM) preserved?

- **Ecchymosis:** Is there evidence of trauma? Does the patient have any underlying bleeding disorders? If there is no trauma or the mechanism of injury does not fit the presentation, consider ordering a coagulation panel and appropriate workup.
- **Symmetry:** Inspect the contour of the musculature and position.

Palpation

Palpate any areas of tenderness or disability. The cardinal signs of inflammation—tumor, rubor, calor, and dolor (mass, redness, heat, and pain)—should be sought. A focused examination, combined with a good knowledge of anatomy, can greatly narrow the differential diagnosis and limit the use of diagnostic tests. Palpation through the ROM examination also can provide clues. In most cases, percussion is unnecessary, although oncologic bone pain, especially in the spine, can be very sensitive to percussion.

Swelling or effusion can be palpated in most joints, with the notable exception of the hip. The presence of swelling of effusion indicates disease or injury to the joint or surrounding synovial membrane. The presence of crepitus is an obvious indicator that something is wrong. Secondary to trauma, grating crepitus is diagnostic of fracture; without trauma, it can indicate calcific tendonitis, osteoarthritis, old fracture fragments, or heterotopic ossification.

Range and Quality of Motion

A goniometer is a useful and easy means of estimating the patient's ROM. Each chapter in this book provides the appropriate ROM. These should serve as a rough guide for most adults, but normal outliers occur at both ends of the spectrum. The ease and fluidity of this motion can be revealing. Gait is extremely important as well, and it merits its own discussion.

The ROM should be tested both passively and actively, with the results from the affected side being compared with those from the contralateral side. Painful active, but not passive, ranging of motion indicates a muscular component either causing or aggravating the underlying condition.

Strength

Weakness is a good general symptom to report. The magnitude of weakness can be graded according to a commonly used system (Table 1.2).

Table 1.2 Strength Scale

Ranking	Significance
0	No strength; no muscular contraction
1	Muscular contraction is present but ineffective; no movement
2	Very weak motion, dependent on position
3	Movement against gravity is possible; no resistance
4	Movement against gravity; some resistance
5	Full, normal strength

Sensation

As previously noted, the value of knowledge regarding human neurologic anatomy pays off in the localization of signs and symptoms. The cutaneous sensation of orthopaedic patients should be assessed and charted (Table 1.3).

The commonly used methods of testing different modes of sensation are:

- **Proprioception:** Joint position is tested by asking the patient in which direction individual fingers are moved (up or down) with the patient not looking. Repeat for the foot. The Romberg test is useful for identifying central nervous system discrepancies in proprioception.
- **Pain/temperature:** Pain can be tested by several methods according to the patient's level of function. A sternal rub should be reserved for patients suspected of coma. Test temperature using the cool steel of the reflex hammer on bilateral skin. For instance, testing of

Table 1.3 Sensory Examination

Description	Significance
Absent	Associated with complete nerve transection and loss of all aspects of nerve function
Deep pain	Severe injury, comatose
Localizes/protective sensation	Proprioception intact
Sensitive to light touch	Good screening assessment; if intact, likely normal

diabetic neuropathy may reveal symmetric, "stocking-and-glove" pattern insensitivity to the bilateral lower extremities.

- **Stereognosis:** Ask the patient to identify a coin in each hand without looking (e.g., "a quarter").
- **Graphesthesia:** Trace a "figure-eight" on the skin bilaterally, and ask what shape is being made.

Note: Always test the affected side, and then compare your findings with those of the opposite side.

Reflexes

Reflexes should also be checked, because they localize to their corresponding spinal level. They can be characterized using the rating system given in Table 1.4.

If weak reflexes are elicited or exaggerated and the examiner is unsure if they are caused by a distracted patient or other factors, it is necessary to perform a **Jendrassik maneuver.** Ask the patient to tonically contract muscle groups that are not directly involved, thereby reinforcing a weak reflex and distracting conscious inhibition of the reflex. For example, have the patient pull against his or her own grip while testing a patellar reflex or press down on the examination table with the legs while testing a biceps reflex.

If the complexity of the examination excludes simple localization, use of electromyelography is beneficial (Table 1.5).

Referral to or consultation with a neurologist can confirm if adequate conduction is present or if muscle denervation or other pathologies exist (Table 1.6).

Nerve injuries often are encountered in trauma and during planned procedures. The most common complaint occurs when the nerve is traumatized, but not physically crushed or severed (i.e., manipulation with retractors), and conduction is disrupted, which results in a **neurapraxia.** The natural course of a neurapraxia is gradual return

Table 1.4 Grading of Reflexes

Grade	Response
0+	Absent
1+	Hypoactive
2+	Normal
3+	Brisk
4+	Hyperactive with clonus

Table 1.5 Indications for Electromyelography

Muscle dysfunction

Suspected cervical radiculopathy

Carpal tunnel syndrome

Sciatic nerve pathology

Muscle weakness

Muscle atrophy

Abnormal cutaneous sensation

Malingering

Brachial plexopathy

Neuronopathy (amyotrophic lateral sclerosis)

Pain disorder

of function and sensation over several weeks to several months. Greater degree of injury can damage the nerve enough to delay or prevent any recovery at all, which is termed **axonotmesis.** Complete severance of a nerve (**neurotmesis**) can lead to permanent paralysis/loss of function without surgical repair.

RADIOGRAPHIC EVALUATION

Interpretation of Radiographs

Skeletal radiographs commonly are ordered when the complaint (pain/deformity) coincides with the occurrence of trauma or long-standing joint pain. A radiograph surely would be useful in a myriad of other sce-

Table 1.6 Common Nerve Injuries Associated with Orthopaedic Trauma

Nerve	Associated Trauma
Axillary	Dislocated shoulder
Median/ulnar	Supracondylar humerus, elbow fracture/dislocation
Sciatic	Acetabular fracture/surgical misadventure
Femoral	Dislocated hip
Tibial/fibular	Tibial plateau, supracondylar knee
Cauda equina	Sacral fracture

narios, but they rarely are obtained when a clinician is "fishing" for a diagnosis. Unnecessary exposure to x-rays is not popular among radiologists.

As often as possible, the examination of the radiograph should be **systematic.** The approach should not be so much standardized as it should be methodical (i.e., to match your own priorities and skill level). At the most basic level, "that does not look right" is a perfectly acceptable reaction for someone who has a few "normals" under his or her belt but is lacking the knowledge to diagnose specifics. Resist jumping to a conclusion about discerning an obvious deformity and disturbing the routine that you have established. The satisfaction of finding a sought-after deformity in a radiograph distracts a person without a system from seeing additional findings on the image—even ones outside of your specialty. Fortunately, skeletal radiographs are always accompanied by a history and physical examination, which in many cases are performed in anticipation of a particular diagnosis. **ABC'S** is a helpful mnemonic for approaching and interpreting an x-ray:

Alignment
Bone (fracture, density, abnormalities, cortices)
Cartilage
Soft tissue

In addition, a high clinical suspicion of fracture based on the mechanism of injury, age, and physical examination, regardless of the radiographic findings, should be managed as a fracture with appropriate rest and immobilization. Follow-up radiographs can be performed between 1 and 2 weeks later and may reveal osteoblastic fracture repair, resorption, and periosteal reaction as a bony callous.

Several items should be noted or presented on rounds:

- Determine whether the view is adequate (over- or underpenetration). Note the degree of rotation, whether the "right site/right side" is in view, and especially whether you are viewing the radiograph from the **correct patient.**
- Determine whether you can visualize the joint above and below the site in question in this radiograph or in the series.
- The conveyance of the anatomic structures being evaluated is very helpful to the audience—and to yourself. This provides reassurance that the pertinent structures are visible. Knowledge of normal anatomy and alignment is extremely helpful; however, "I don't know what this thing is" is a perfectly acceptable statement to utter while reading a radiograph.
- In reading the radiograph, pay attention to the margin of all bony cortices, and look for any disruption that may indicate a fracture.

- Scrutinize articular surfaces for involvement in a fracture pattern as well as for widening or narrowing of the joint. The presence of a fat and/or fluid level in a joint space is nearly pathognomonic for an articular fracture.
- Study the surrounding soft tissue for the presence of swelling, air (cellulitis or osteomyelitis), bony fragments, or fat pad enlargement. In the elbow, an increased anterior region (the anterior fat pad), **especially the posterior fat pads,** often indicates a fracture (Fig. 1.1).

Fracture

Students and nonradiologists do not need to provide interpretations of magnetic resonance imaging (MRI) results or skeletal scintigraphy, but they often are called on to accurately interpret radiographs and to describe fractures. Common descriptors of fractures include transverse, oblique, spiral, and simple or comminuted. Additional descriptors include **complete/incomplete, impacted, pathological,** and **avulsion** (Table 1.7).

Other items to note regarding fractures include:

- It is important to note whether the fracture involves the joint (i.e., is **intra-articular**).
- **Angulation** is judged in terms of direction (medial/lateral or varus/valgus) or the number of degrees by which the fracture fragment is directed from the long axis of the bone in question. The most proximal segment of bone to the fracture is used to judge angulation of the distal fragment.
- **Displacement** is judged by the direction in which a fracture fragment has moved in anteroposterior or mediolateral planes. The amount of movement is given in units such as centimeters.
- Skeletal radiographs should include a minimum of two views, taken 90° to one another, to evaluate a three-dimensional structure.

Figure 1.2 is an anteroposterior view of the right hip in a skeletally mature 18-year-old with good penetration and without significant rotation. A basic approach to the anteroposterior of the right hip, as shown here, could consist of the following:

1. Shenton's line, which coincides with the left hip, is intact, and the articular surface of the acetabulum appears to be normal in this view.
2. Following the cortical margins from the femoral shaft over the greater trochanter and along the femoral neck gives an intact appearance without disruption. The same can be said of the

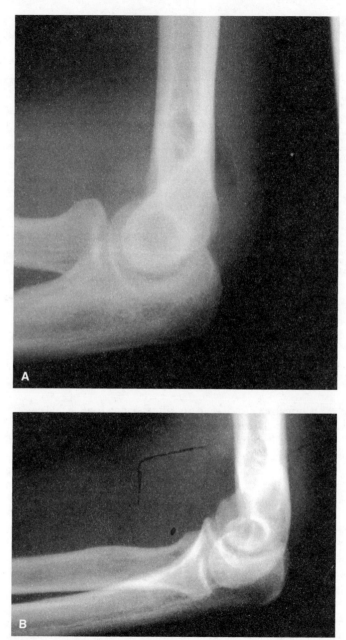

Figure 1.1 a: Radiograph showing the posterior fat pad. **b:** Radiograph showing the anterior fat pad.

Table 1.7 Fracture Patterns

Pattern	Description
Open fracture	Overlying skin not intact
Complete	Both cortices disrupted
Incomplete	Only one cortex disrupted
Transverse	Right angle to the long axis of the shaft
Oblique	At an angle to the shaft
Spiral	Via a torsional injury, spiral pattern, sharp fragments
Comminuted	More than two fragments
Segmental	Comminuted but two large fragments, often from transverse fractures
Butterfly	Triangular floating segment

inferior aspect of the neck extending along the lesser trochanter and medial shaft.
3. The femoral head appears to be intact and without evidence of joint erosion, fracture, or sclerosis.
4. Evaluating the soft tissue structures proximal to the hip reveals no obvious deformities or abnormalities.

Abnormal findings deviate from the above and one should describe what is seen. In the case of a fracture, some basic description precedes the advanced description of common fracture patterns, degree of osteopenia or sclerosis, and classification scheme or "zebra" finding. A few other pertinent descriptive terms include *stress*, *pathological*, *fatigue*, or *neuropathic* (Table 1.8). Table 1.9 presents a glossary of radiologic fracture terms.

A neuropathic injury is one that results from long-standing diabetes and other etiologies (e.g., postinfectious neuropathy or syrinx) and causes abnormal wear in the joint, fractures, or dislocations. It is marked by degeneration of the bone and joint, destruction of the bone, sclerosis, disorganized new bone growth, and loose bodies. A **Charcot joint** is the term that is given to such a joint.

Radiographic indicators of osteoarthritis include joint space narrowing, osteophytes, subchondral sclerosis, and subchondral cysts. Weight-bearing radiographs are indicated in the evaluation of osteoarthritis.

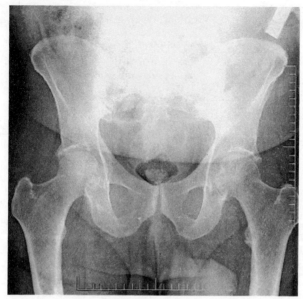

Figure 1.2 Anteroposterior radiograph of a normal hip.

OTHER IMAGING MODALITIES

Other imaging modalities include computed tomography (CT), MRI, and radioisotope imaging. Instructions for ordering medical imaging studies are given in Table 1.10.

Computed Tomography

Computed tomography—or, as a radiology attending of mine calls it, "the truth machine"—is a very accurate means of evaluating the musculoskeletal system. The sensitivity and specificity of CT are much

Table 1.8 Explanatory Terms Used to Describe Fractures

Term	Description
Stress fracture	If the fracture results from chronically applied force to the bone
Pathological fracture	If the underlying bone is diseased
Insufficiency fracture	If the underlying bone is osteopenic
Fatigue fracture	If the underlying bone is normal

Table 1.9 Glossary of Radiologic Fractures

Term	Description
Osteochondral fracture	Fracture of cartilaginous surface of the bone, such as in Hill-Sachs fractures
Stable fracture	Good apposition of fracture fragments
Complete fracture	Involves both cortices
Incomplete fracture	Disruption of only one cortex
Unstable fracture	Poorly oriented fracture fragments; will not heal correctly on their own or in a cast; usually requires open reduction with internal fixation
Loose body	Old fracture fragment (bone or cartilage; also called joint mice if articular)
Occult fracture	A fracture not accompanied by easily discernible signs or symptoms
Avulsion fracture	Fracture of the bony attachment of a muscle by muscular contraction or trauma
Subluxation	Partial loss of normal articular continuity
Dislocation	Corresponding joint surfaces no longer congruent
Distraction	Opposing ends of a fracture are pulled apart
Impaction	Fracture with the two fragments driven together end to end
Comminuted fracture	Multiple fracture fragments present
Varus angulation	Deviating away from the midline
Valgus angulation	Deviating toward the midline
Angulation	Deviation from normal bone alignment; the direction of angulation is derived from the apex of the angle created by the two fragments
Displacement	Anteroposterior or mediolateral translation of a fracture fragment in relation to the proximal fragment
Stress fracture	Fracture resulting from chronically applied force to the bone
Pathological fracture	Underlying bone is diseased (e.g., tumor)
Insufficiency fracture	Underlying bone is osteopenic
Fatigue fracture	Fracture of normal bone subjected to abnormal stresses

Table 1.10 Instructions for Ordering Medical Imaging Studies

Individual radiology departments perform standard views based on what site is to be examined. The following information should be included with all orders for imaging studies:

- Site to be examined, and radiography, CT, MRI, or other imaging to be provided.
- Nonstandard views (e.g., ulnar deviation view for scaphoid fracture; in some cases, these views are also standard).
- Location of physical complaint (e.g., painful wrist).
- History (radiologists are physicians, after all, and benefit from a good history).
- Clinical suspicion is optional (e.g., to rule out osteomyelitis).

better than with plain-film radiography, especially for subtle fracture lines. The cost-effectiveness of routine CT scanning, however, makes it somewhat prohibitive as anything but an advanced study. Computed tomography often is invoked when clinical suspicion is high but radiographic findings are low or difficult to interpret. Subtle cortical fractures are seen in better detail, but these fractures are usually not treated any differently than if only suspected on plain-film radiographs. The major role of CT in orthopaedics is in the evaluation of complex structures, such as the spine, face, shoulder complex, hip, pelvis, knee, tibial plateau, and sometimes, the foot. This modality is essential in the evaluation of pelvic and acetabular fractures because of their complexity and the need for preoperative planning. Additional benefits of CT include the ability to obtain multiple planar views without manipulating the injured patient, speed (in contrast to MRI), and the now-increasing availability of three-dimensional reconstructions. In addition, digital subtraction software has made it possible to remove overlying soft tissue so that only bony or vascular structures are portrayed in these reconstructions.

Magnetic Resonance Imaging

Magnetic resonance imaging was once prohibitively expensive, and its role in the evaluation of orthopaedic injuries and pathology was unclear. Today, however, MRI has emerged as the gold standard for soft tissue imaging.

Because MRI does not involve radiation, it is safer than CT. Very strong magnets are used to briefly disturb hydrogen atoms, and the radiowaves given off by these perturbations are sensed and

Table 1.11 Technetium-99 (Tc99m) Isotopes Used in Nuclear Imaging

Isotope	Site of Uptake
Tc99m-pertechnetate	Thyroid
Tc99m-macroaggregated albumin	Pulmonary capillaries
Tc99m-methylene diphosphate	Bone

interpreted by the scanner. The concept of signal intensity is more appropriate than radiolucency/density, and the intensity of the signal is dependent on the concentration of hydrogen atoms, which is preset. The highest concentration (and, therefore, the greater intensity) is found in hydrogen-rich tissue, such as fat, and in water.

Compared with CT, MRI does not show fractures as well, is more time-intensive, and last but not least, is more costly. Because of the longer data acquisition time required, motion artifact is more of a problem as well.

The MRI data sets can be organized into multiple modalities, two of which are T_1- or T_2-weighted images. Compact bone has low signal intensity in both and appears dark. Fat appears brighter in T_1- than T_2-weighted images because of its water content and, therefore, increased signal intensity.

Radioisotope Imaging

Technetium-99 (Tc99m) is a radionuclide that is preferentially taken up by certain tissues when introduced into the body by intravenous injection. Three Tc99m isotopes are used in nuclear imaging (Table 1.11); of these, Tc99m-methylene diphosphate is readily taken up by bone.

Bone scanning portrays the degree of bone cell uptake of the tracer and, therefore, the amount of cell turnover in bone. These areas appear dark, and they can indicate abnormal bone growth in the analysis of cancer metastasis or osteomyelitis.

2

Cervical Spine

The full spine with primary and secondary curves is shown in Figure 2.1. The three-column model of the spine is shown in Figure 2.2.

ANATOMY

The cervical spine includes seven cervical vertebrae (typical vertebrae) (Figs. 2.3 and 2.4). These cervical vertebrae include the following structures:

Articular facets: Two superior and two inferior facets articulate with the vertebrae above and below it; these are termed zygapophyseal joints.

Body (centrum): Mass of the vertebrae; along with the disk, it supports the weight of the skull.

C1 atlas (Fig. 2.5): Ring structure; no body, no spinous process; cradles the occipital condyles; atlanto-occipital joint permits approximately 10–15° of flexion/extension.

C2 axis (Fig. 2.5): Odontoid process (dens) is an anatomic restraint and pivot for the atlas; it has the smallest transverse processes of all vertebrae and a bifid spinous process.

C7 (vertebra prominens): Site of attachment of ligamentum nuchae; longest spinous process of the column.

Laminae: Extend from the pedicles and fuse with each other at the spinous process.

Pedicles: Form the base of the vertebral arch bilaterally.

Spinous processes: Posterior projection; C7 has the largest process.

Transverse foramina: Arise at C6 and transmit the vertebral artery into the basal skull.

Transverse processes: Arise from the lateral aspects of the vertebral arches between the pedicle and lamina.

Upper cervical ligaments: Include the cruciform ligament and the alar ligaments, which help anchor the dens against the

15

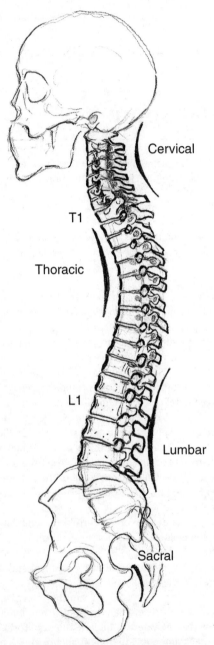

Figure 2.1 Full spine, with primary and secondary curves.

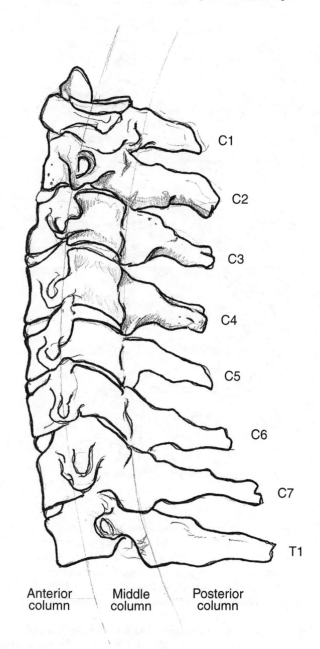

C1

C2

C3

C4

C5

C6

C7

T1

Anterior
column

Middle
column

Posterior
column

Figure 2.2 Three-column model of the spine.

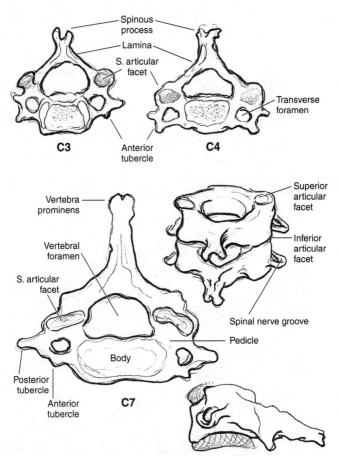

Figure 2.3 C3 to C7 (typical vertebrae). S., superior.

posterior aspect of the anterior arch of the atlas. The anterior and atlanto-occipital ligaments (uppermost anterior longitudinal ligament) anchor C1 with the foramen magnum, and the anterior atlantoaxial ligament secures C1 to C2. The upper segment of the posterior longitudinal ligament becomes the tectorial membrane and attaches at the anterior foramen magnum.

Vertebral canal (neuroforamina): Formed by the body (anteriorly), paired lamina (laterally), and spinous process (posteriorly); contains the spinal cord.

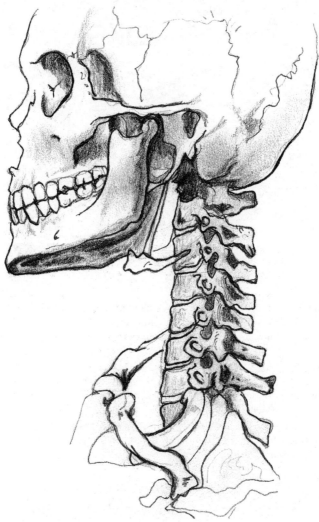

Figure 2.4 Cervical spine. Note that the foramen of the vertebral artery arises at C6.

BASIC EXAMINATION

Assessment of the cervical spine should always begin with basic patient history, observation, and palpation of pertinent structures. Neurologic examination should precede a physical examination. Pay special

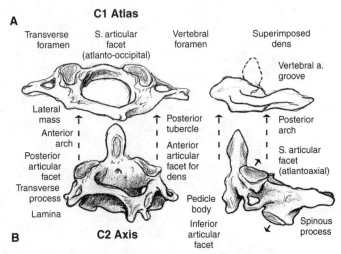

Figure 2.5 a: C1 atlas. **b:** C2 axis. a., artery; S., superior.

attention to bony deformities, such as step-offs and spinous process fractures. Obvious neck muscle tension also can guide the direction of the assessment, and the nature and direction of pain can be valuable if the pain is obviously in a peripheral nerve or dermatomal distribution. The high-yield tests for the cervical spine include cervical root assessment using the biceps, triceps, and brachioradialis reflexes. Assessment of brachial plexus derivatives is performed in association with the following peripheral nerves: radial, ulnar, median, and musculocutaneous. Motor function is assessed quickly with the tests/actions listed in Table 2.1, whereas sensation is assessed according to the cutaneous and spinal dermatomes (Fig. 2.6).

Table 2.1 Brachial Plexus Derivatives and Their Actions

Brachial Plexus Derivative	Action
Radial nerve	Wrist and thumb extension
Ulnar nerve	Abduction (little finger)
Median nerve	Thumb pinch, opposition of thumb, thumb abduction
Axillary nerve	Deltoid
Musculocutaneous nerve	Biceps

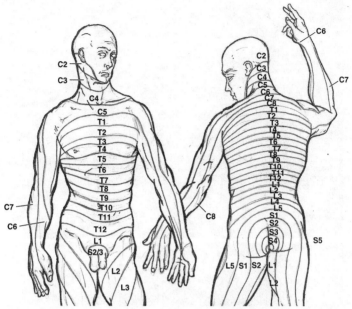

Figure 2.6 Cervical dermatomes. The anatomic correlations to the cervical nerve roots are invaluable in the physical diagnosis of impingement, traumatic deficit, and neuropathic symptoms.

Once spinal cord trauma has been ruled out, the neck and shoulder joint complex can be taken through its full range of motion:

Flexion	45°
Extension	55°
Lateral motion	40°
Rotary motion	70°

Specialized tests can be included to narrow the focus of the examination and to aid in the localization of a lesion:

- 50% of flexion and extension occurs between the occiput and C1, and the remaining is distributed from C2 to C7 (especially C5 and C6).
- 50% of rotation is between C1 and C2, and the remaining is distributed from C2 to C7.

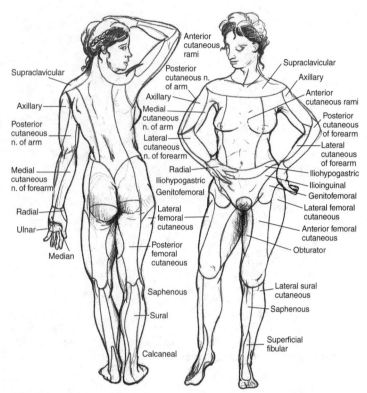

Figure 2.7 Cutaneous distribution of sensory nerves.

Palpation

Palpation of soft tissue structures aids in the localization of cervical spine tenderness or other abnormal findings (Table 2.2). Also palpate the occiput, inion, superior nuchal line, mastoid processes, spinous processes of cervical vertebrae, and facet joints:

Table 2.2 Correlation Between Anatomic Structure and Cervical Vertebrae

Anatomic Structure	Cervical Correlation
Hyoid	C3
Thyroid cartilage	C4 and C5
First cricoid cartilage	C6

- Facet joints at C5 and C6 are the most often injured or dislocated.
- Palpate for the presence of a cervical rib, which can be a setup for vascular and neurologic pathology.

  Palpation of soft tissue structures includes:

- **Anterior triangle** (defined laterally by the sternocleidomastoids [two heads], superiorly by the mandible, and inferiorly by the suprasternal notch): Lymph node chain, thyroid, carotid pulse, parotid, and supraclavicular fossa.
- **Posterior triangle:** Trapezius, lymph nodes (posterior chain), greater occipital nodes, and superior nuchal ligament.

Muscle Testing

The prime muscles involved in movement of the neck are listed in Table 2.3. Sensory distribution (Figure 2.7) via cervical roots follows this pattern:

- **C5:** Lateral arm, axillary nerve;
- **C6:** Lateral forearm, thumb, index, and half of middle finger, sensory branches of the musculocutaneous nerve;
- **C7:** Middle finger;
- **C8:** Ring and little finger, medial forearm, medial antebrachial cutaneous nerve;
- **T1:** Medial arm, medial antebrachial cutaneous nerve.

  Figure 2.8 shows the distribution of the brachial plexus, and Figure 2.9 shows the motor levels that correspond to the reflexes.

Table 2.3 Muscular Motion of the Cervical Spine

	Flexion	Extension	Lateral Rotation	Lateral Bending
Primary	Sternocleido-mastoid (cranial nerve XI)	1. Paravertebral extensors (splenius, capitis, and semispinalis) 2. Trapezius (cranial nerve XI)	Sternoclei-domastoid	Scalenus anticus, medius, and posticus
Secondary	1. Scalenus 2. Prevertebral muscles	Various small intrinsic muscles of the neck	Small intrinsic muscles of the neck	Small intrinsic muscles of the neck

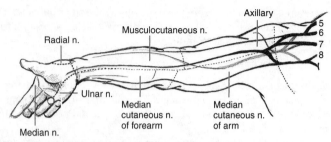

Figure 2.8 Distribution of the brachial plexus. n., nerve.

Table 2.4 presents information regarding the upper extremity reflex corollaries, and Table 2.5 lists the major peripheral nerves and summarizes how to evaluate them. Figure 2.10 correlates with Table 2.5.

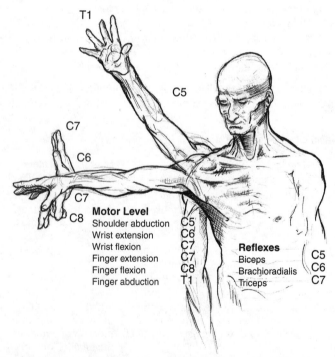

Motor Level		
Shoulder abduction	C5	
Wrist extension	C6	
Wrist flexion	C7	
Finger extension	C7	**Reflexes**
Finger flexion	C8	Biceps C5
Finger abduction	T1	Brachioradialis C6
		Triceps C7

Figure 2.9 Motor levels and reflexes corresponding to cervical level.

Table 2.4 Upper Extremity Reflex Corollaries

Reflex	Disk	Root	Muscle	Sensation	Nerve
Biceps	C4 and C5	C5	Deltoid, biceps	Lateral arm • Lateral deltoid area is almost pure C5	Axillary, musculocutaneous
Brachioradialis	C5 and C6	C6	**Wrist extensors group** 1. Extensor carpi radialis longus 2. Extensor carpi radialis brevis 3. Extensor carpi ulnaris **Biceps**	Lateral forearm, musculocutaneous	Radial Musculocutaneous
Triceps	C6 and C7	C7	**Wrist flexor group** 1. Flexor carpi radialis 2. Flexor carpi ulnaris **Finger flexors** 1. Extensor digitorum communis 2. Extensor digitorum indicis 3. Extensor digitorum minimi **Triceps**	Middle finger	Median, ulnar Radial Radial
	C7 and T1	C8	**Finger flexors** 1. Flexor digitorum superficialis 2. Flexor digitorum profundus **Hand intrinsics**	Medial forearm, medial antebrachial cutaneous	Median Ulnar and median
	T1 and T2	T1	**Hand intrinsics** 1. Dorsal interossei 2. Abductor digiti quinti	Medial arm, median brachial cutaneous	Ulnar

Table 2.5 Major Peripheral Nerves

Nerve	Motor Test	Sensation Test
Radial nerve	Wrist and thumb extension	Dorsal web space between thumb and index finger
Ulnar nerve	Abduction (little finger)	Distal aspect of little finger
Median nerve	Thumb pinch, opposition of thumb, thumb abduction	Distal radial aspect of index finger
Axillary nerve	Deltoid	Lateral arm, pure deltoid patch
Musculocutaneous nerve	Biceps	Lateral forearm

SPECIAL TESTS

Note: Many of these tests are not indicated in the setting of cervical spinal trauma.

Adson's Test

The Adson's test (Fig. 2.11) indicates occlusion of the subclavian by the scalenes and/or a cervical rib. Feel the radial pulse while abducting, extending, and externally rotating the humerus.

Ankle Clonus

Quickly dorsiflex the foot while cradling the heel in the palm to relieve the load. A positive test is a multiple-beat clonus, which strongly suggests an upper motor neuron lesion of the spinal cord or brain.

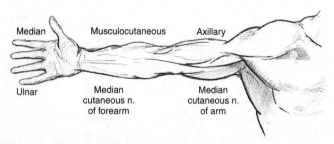

Figure 2.10 Major peripheral nerves. n., nerve.

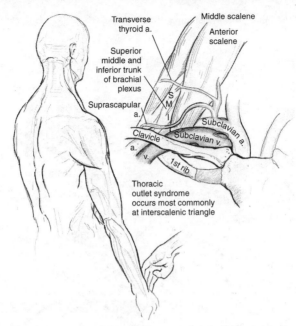

Figure 2.11 Adson's test. Abduct arm in extension; feel pulse while externally rotating a., artery; I, inferior; M, middle; S, superior; v., vein.

Bakody sign

The Bakody sign indicates a cervical radiculopathy. The patient raises a hand on top of the head. A positive test is a reduction of pain and a relief of tension on the nerve roots, sensory nerves, and brachial plexus.

Compression/Distraction

The compression/distraction test (Fig. 2.12) involves:

- **Compression:** Push down on the skull of the seated patient. If pain from neural foramen stenosis exists, then this movement will cause neck or extremity pain. This should be a gentle maneuver and does not come completely without risk or liability.
- **Distraction:** Pull traction up on skull of the seated patient. If cervical or extremity pain is relieved, then it is likely caused by neural foramina compression.

Doorbell Sign

The doorbell sign (Fig. 2.13) indicates nerve root tension/radiculopathy. Deep palpation of the C5 segment produces pain in the superior scapulovertebral border that radiates down the arm. Positive local pain indicates a cervical sprain/strain.

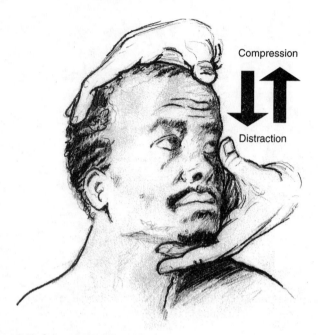

Compression

Distraction

Figure 2.12 Compression/distraction.

Halstead Maneuver

The Halstead maneuver (Fig. 2.14) shows neurovascular compression. In a seated patient, palpate a radial pulse, and then pull traction on the patient's arm downward while the patient extends his or her head backward. A positive test is the reproduction of symptoms such as paresthesias, which indicate thoracic outlet syndrome, a cervical rib, or anterior scalene syndrome.

Hoffmann's Sign

The myelopathic Hoffman's sign (Fig. 2.15) indicates an upper motor neuron lesion, such as multiple sclerosis, a spinal cord tumor, compression, or traumatic spondylosis. Flick the distal interphalangeal (DIP) joint of the long finger. A positive test is involuntary flexion of the DIP joint of the thumb and index finger.

Jackson's Compression

Jackson's compression (Fig. 2.16) indicates nerve involvement from a space-occupying lesion, subluxation, inflammation, degenerative joint

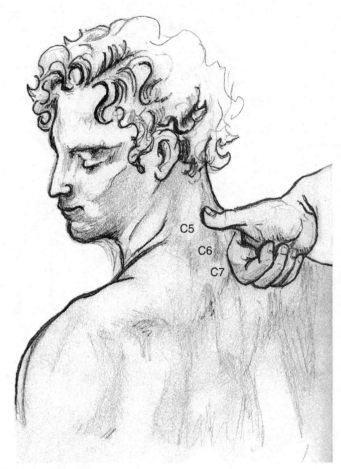

Figure 2.13 Doorbell sign.

disease, tumor, or disk herniation. Apply downward pressure on the seated patient's head, with the head bent obliquely backward. A positive test is localized pain that radiates down the arm.

Lhermitte's Sign

Lhermitte's sign (Fig. 2.17) indicates spinal canal stenosis, multiple sclerosis, cervical disk impingement, or tumor. A positive test is forward flexion of the neck causing an electrical, shooting pain down the spinal cord; this is similar to radicular sciatic pain. **A true positive**

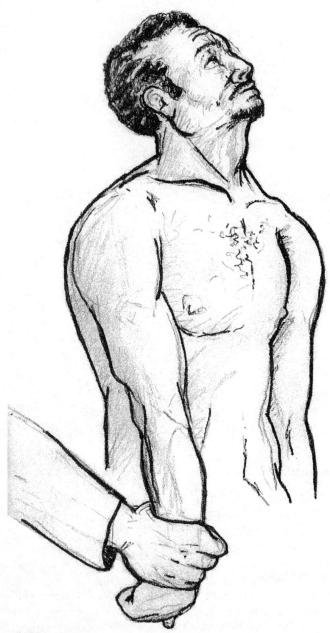

Figure 2.14 Halstead maneuver.

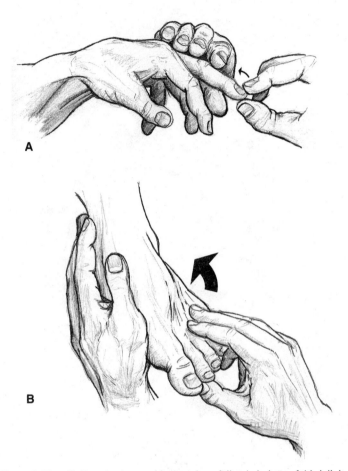

Figure 2.15 a: Hoffman's sign; rapid extension of distal phalanx of third digit. **b:** Ankle clonus.

Lhermitte's sign should be taken very seriously, and it encompasses a serious differential diagnosis. A positive test is most commonly encountered in patients with multiple sclerosis via cervical spinal cord demyelination. The patient with multiple sclerosis also characteristically presents with ulnar nerve distribution paresthesias and visual changes reflecting optic neuritis. The differential diagnosis includes traumatic or compressive myelopathy (e.g., cervical spondylosis and epidural, subdural, and intraparenchymatous tumors),

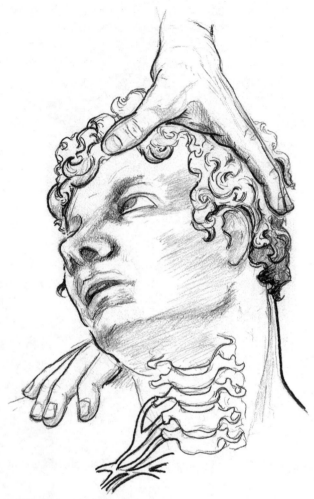

Figure 2.16 Jackson's compression.

radiation myelitis, pernicious anemia (subacute combined degeneration), Behçet's disease, and systemic lupus erythematosus.

Rust's Sign

A patient holding the weight of the head in the hands or lifting the head manually when arising from lying down is a positive Rust's sign, which

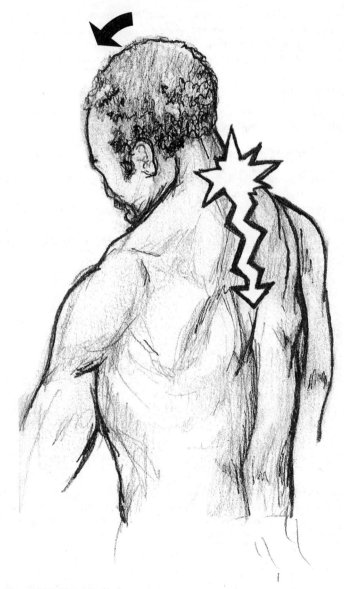

Figure 2.17 Lhermitte's sign.

indicates a severe sprain, rheumatoid arthritis, fracture, or severe cervical subluxation. If the result is positive, no further active or passive testing is necessary. Perform anteroposterior (AP), lateral, and odontoid imaging immediately, and place a cervical collar on the patient.

Swallowing

Dysphagia, which is exacerbated with a forced swallow, can indicate anterior cervical spine swelling.

Valsalva Test

Increased pain when bearing down can indicate a bulging or herniated disk (i.e., radicular symptom).

Note: Use caution in patients who are prone to syncope.

RADIOLOGIC APPROACH TO THE CERVICAL SPINE
Trauma

The frequency of cervical vertebrae injury with trauma is:

- **Motor-vehicle accident:** 1st > 5th > 6th > 7th cervical vertebrae.
- **Posttraumatic fall:** 5th > 6th > 7th cervical vertebrae.

When evaluating a patient with spinal trauma and neurologic deficits or any sudden onset of neurologic symptoms, the decision to perform magnetic resonance imaging should be swift. Early treatment with intravenous steroids has produced considerable decreases in morbidity in cases of spinal cord contusion and hematomas; these may occur in the absence of occult fractures and need quick recognition and treatment.

Clearing the Cervical Spine

Clearing the cervical spine is an important and ubiquitous task. Before assessment, you must be presented with an oriented patient (e.g., aware of person, place, and time) with no distracting injuries (i.e., femur fracture or burns) and no intoxicants.

Views

The three primary views to obtain in cervical spine trauma are the AP, lateral, and odontoid. Some radiology departments also include an oblique view and swimmer's view for a total of five views, but three views is a minimum requirement. In trauma centers, five views is the standard.

The full cervical spine from occiput to T1 must be well visualized in an alert patient. A raised arm "swimmer's view" is necessary if the body of T1 is not visible on the standard lateral radiograph.

If pain persists in a patient who has negative standard radiographs, flexion and extension views can be obtained. Because of its sensitivity, however, computed tomography (CT) is more commonly performed in emergency departments. The rules change for altered level of consciousness or comatose patients who all merit a CT to rule out fracture. Patients should be left in a cervical collar until a definitive "rule out" is made.

It is important to note that the sensitivity of plain-film radiographs for "ruling out" cervical spine injuries is not very high. In a retrospective analysis published by the *Journal of Trauma* in 1993, Woodring and Lee compared plain-film radiographs to CT scans, and those authors found that "prospectively, the trauma series improved the sensitivity of plain-film radiographs for detecting cervical injuries but still did not detect 61% of the fractures and 36% of the subluxations and dislocations, and falsely identified 23% of the patients, half of whom had unstable cervical injuries, as having normal cervical spines." Plain-film radiographs have an average reported sensitivity of 40–60%, whereas helical CT has a reported sensitivity and specificity in the high 90s. This underscores the value of a good prehospital report from paramedics detailing the mechanism of injury. When the index of suspicion is high, CT is a better choice.

Note: Check to make sure you have the correct patient, the correct date, and the correct anatomy.

Anteroposterior View

An AP view (Fig. 2.18) is a good view of C3 to C7. **Adequate views show no rotation or angular tilt.** Spinous processes should be midline and are evenly spaced. Evaluate the lateral masses for compression fractures (e.g., pie-shaped body or lateral displacement). The lateral margins should be smooth and continuous.

Note equal separation of the spinous processes in the midline to evaluate for flexion injuries. In patients with any rotation of spinous processes or a distance greater than 1.5-fold the interspinous distance above or below, obtain an oblique view to assess for subluxation/dislocation/facet fracture.

The AP view is best for vertical compression fractures. These fractures show a sagittally oriented fracture extending from end plate to end plate.

The fibrocartilaginous disk spaces should be equal.

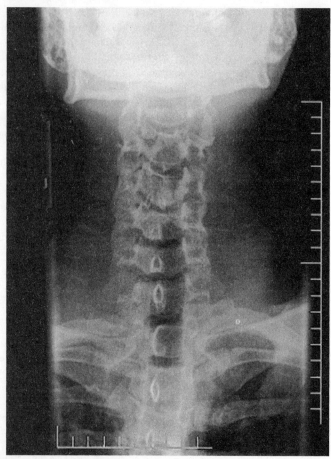

Figure 2.18 Anteroposterior radiograph of the cervical spine.

Lateral View

An adequate lateral view (Fig. 2.19) shows the lateral spine from the basilar skull to the cervicothoracic junction. If possible, identify the following:

- Each cervical vertebra.
- Cartilaginous disk spaces.
- Four cervical lordotic curves.
- C2 neural arch (Hangman's fracture).
- Laminae, spinous processes, lateral masses, and articular facets.

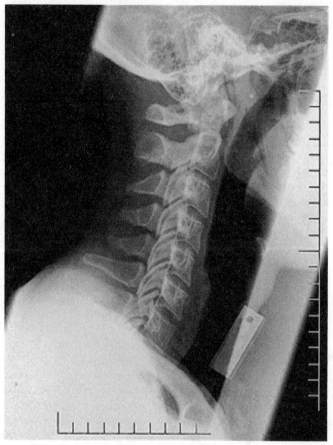

Figure 2.19 Lateral radiograph of the cervical spine.

Key relationships in the evaluation of the lateral view include:

- **Atlantoaxial distance** (atlantodental interval).
  - **Children** (<10 years): <3.5 mm;
  - **Adults:** <3 mm.
  Note: A C1-on-C2 anterior shift of more than 3–5 mm implies injury to the transverse ligament and is termed **atlantoaxial subluxation.** This interval should be scrutinized in all children with Down syndrome and in patients with rheumatoid arthritis who have an increased risk. A shift of more than 5 mm implies disruption of the alar ligaments as well.

- **Horizontal alignment:** Best measured by the posterior cortices.
  - **Translation** (anterior or posterior): >3.5 mm is unstable.
  - **Facet fracture:** <25% relative shift of one vertebral body over the other.
  - **Facet dislocation** (unilateral or bilateral): 25% to >50% relative shift;
- **Vertebral body translation:** Patterns of instability include:
  - 1.7 mm of disk widening, or 3.5 mm of translational displacement (measure from the inferior end plates).
  - 11° of angulation compared with contiguous cervical vertebrae.
- **Soft tissue structures:** Especially the prevertebral space, which can average 5–10 mm down to the level of C4. After C4, however, this distance can vary widely. Focal enlargement of this space can indicate trauma, mass, and abscess. Specific measurements are unnecessary, but the overall contour of the soft tissue contiguous with the cervical vertebrae should be smooth.

Swimmer's View

If the visualization of C7 and T1 is inadequate, then a swimmer's view (i.e., with the arms elevated above the head) should be taken to remove the obstruction by the humerus.

Odontoid View

The odontoid view (Figs. 2.20 and 2.21) is most important in evaluating C1, C2, and the odontoid process (dens). Knowledge of normal variants is helpful, because the appearance of the dens may vary from absent, to hypoplastic, to incompletely fused, and to unfused. This view should be scrutinized in children with Down syndrome and in patients with rheumatoid arthritis; these patients are prone to atlantoaxial subluxation. Adequate radiographs should have no overlap by the basilar skull or teeth, and spinous processes should be in the midline.

If possible, identify the following:

- Odontoid process (dens).
- C2 vertebral body.
- Lateral masses of C1.
- Atlas burst fractures (Jefferson's fracture; are assessed for with this view).
- Displacement of the lateral masses (>7 mm implies disruption of the transverse ligament).
- Progression of disease in rheumatoid arthritis (performed by evaluating the dens and lateral processes).

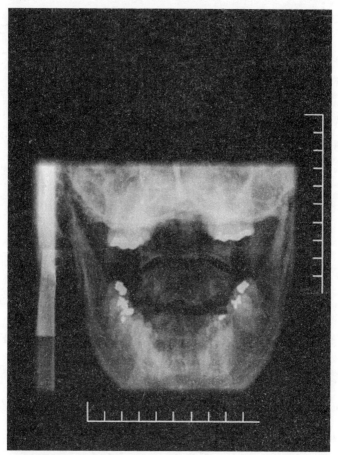

Figure 2.20 Odontoid radiograph (open mouth).

SELECTED FRACTURES AND DISLOCATIONS OF THE CERVICAL SPINE

Facet Dislocation

A unilateral or bilateral facet dislocation involves the anterior displacement of one or both vertebral facet joints, most often because of rotational flexion trauma. Anterior subluxation of a superior vertebra implies facet dislocation, and the degree of the anterior displacement can be used to determine unilateral or bilateral dislocation. If the amount of movement is less than the inferior dislocated vertebrae, then

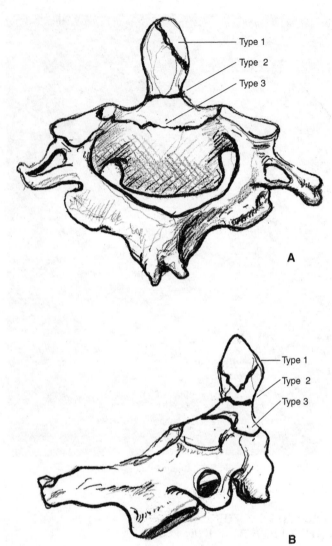

Figure 2.21 Odontoid radiograph of the cervical spine.

this is probably a unilateral injury. More than 50% forward translation, however, necessitates a bilateral dislocation. Lateral radiographs are the most useful in establishing the diagnosis. Treatment can be conservative, involving immobilization with a cervical collar or halo for six weeks or more. Open reduction and internal fixation appear to have good clinical results but require a skilled, specialty orthopedist.

Clay Shoveler's Fracture

The clay shoveler's fracture belongs to the hyperflexion class of cervical spine injuries and is an avulsion/spinous process fatigue fracture, usually at the base of C7 (relative incidence, C7 > C6 > T1). It received its name from early twentieth-century laborers who were prone to this pathology. Intact posterior ligaments make this a stable fracture. Treatment usually consists of applying a hard cervical collar for several weeks, until a bony callous is well developed.

Jefferson's (Burst) Fracture

A Jefferson's fracture involves a fracture of the bilateral C1 arches. Because the C1 vertebra is a closed ring, a traumatic break always involves more than one fracture. The mechanism of both Jefferson's and burst fractures usually is an axial loading/compression type. The Jefferson's fracture is best seen on the odontoid view as the displacement of C1 lateral masses; this often involves a fracture of the dens and disruption of the transverse odontoid ligament. Vertebral artery injuries have been reported, especially with atlanto-occipital dislocations.

These are very unstable fractures, because the main structural support at the occipital condyles is lost. A burst fracture is seen on the AP radiograph as a vertical fracture of the body of the lower cervical vertebrae and on the lateral radiograph as a commutation of the body, usually with some retropulsion of the body. Depending on extent of injury, treatment can vary from immobilization with a halo to surgical fusion. Because the atlantoaxial-occipital complex is responsible for a great deal of motion, fusion of these joints can severely restrict future motion. Approximately 50% of flexion and extension occurs between the occiput and C1, with the remaining distributed from C2 to C7 (especially C5/C6). Approximately 50% of rotation occurs between C1 and C2, with the remaining distributed from C2 to C7.

Dens Fracture

Odontoid, or dens, fractures are classified into three groups:

- **Type 1:** Avulsion fractures of the alar ligament where it inserts at the tip of the dens. This can be seen in association with the atlantoaxial rotary subluxation above and can be life-threatening.

- **Type 2:** The most common type, occurring at the base of the dens. Vascular supply is limited to the dens, and a high rate of nonunion accompanies this fracture.
- **Type 3:** Characterized by the extension of the fracture into the body of C2. Posterior displacement of the fragment is most common and can lead to spinal cord injury (incidence, 10%).

Management of type 1 fractures usually involves a surgical orthosis (halo). Type 2 and type 3 fractures require some immobilization with traction.

Hangman's Fracture (Traumatic Spondylolisthesis of C2)

This injury, once associated with hanging, involves bilateral fractures through the pedicles of C2 as a result of a hyperextension injury. Because hangings have fallen out of favor, the most common mechanism of injury is now motor-vehicle accidents. This is not considered to be an unstable fracture unless it is associated with facet dislocation, and it does not often cause neurologic injury because of the wide spinal canal in the superior cervical spine. Incidentally, death by hanging is largely a product of bilateral occlusion of the carotids and suffocation. Management is immobilization via a cervical orthotic brace. This injury pattern involves hyperextension.

SELECTED DISORDERS OF THE CERVICAL SPINE

Atlantoaxial Rotary Subluxation

Atlantoaxial instability (C1–C2 articulation) is a relatively rare condition in patients without a predisposing pathology. With predisposing laxity or malformation of C1 and C2, the risk is approximately 10–20%. Perhaps the most common associated condition is Down syndrome or other pediatric skeletal hypoplasia. Interestingly, the more severe degrees of dislocation or subluxation often result following a viral upper respiratory tract infection, probably related to local inflammatory processes. Children with Down syndrome who have an atlantodental interval of less than 5 mm should avoid contact sports or other risky activities. The diagnosis is dependent on history (predisposing factors), physical examination findings (pain, restricted range of motion, and torticollis), and imaging (radiography and magnetic resonance imaging). Treatment is generally conservative for instability, such as immobilization with a soft collar or halo traction. More significant instability can include surgical fusion of an unstable joint.

Torticollis

Congenital torticollis (or "wry neck") is a condition that is characterized by involuntary contraction of the neck muscles, leading to a
twisted neck presentation in the infant or child. Treatment is directed
at strengthening of these muscles during physical therapy. Most adult
cases (80%), however, are considered to be idiopathic. Before establishing a diagnosis of idiopathic spinal torticollis, considering other
causes, such as infection (cervical osteomyelitis), tumors via a mass
effect, trauma (e.g., occipital condyle fractures), cervical muscle spasm
following a motor-vehicle accident, odontoid fractures, subluxation,
and drug-induced causes (L-dopa and neuroleptics can mimic this).

Quick Look • Cervical Spine

Note: If the patient is taking cervical spine precautions, evaluate
the patient while he or she is in the cervical collar, or remove
the collar while the head is immobilized by a second caregiver:
- **Inspect** skin and trachea, looking for gross deformity.
- **Palpate** down the length of the spinous process, noting
  crepitus, swelling, or step-offs.

If no trauma:
- **Move neck through range of motion.**
  - **Flexion:** Chin to chest, 45°.
  - **Hyperextension:** Head back, 55°.
  - **Lateral bending:** Side to side, 40°.
  - **Axial rotation:** Chin to shoulder, 70°.
- **Muscle testing.**
  - **Trapezius:** Shrug shoulders (cranial nerve XI).
  - **Sternocleidomastoid:** Flexion.
- **Reflex testing:** If neurologic deficits, cervical stenosis, or
  upper motor neuron (UMN)/lower motor neuron (LMN)
  disorder suspected or if the patient is preoperative or post-
  operative.
  - **Biceps, brachioradialis, triceps.**
    - ■ **Absent:** Neuropathy, LMN lesion.
    - ■ **Hyperactive:** UMN lesion.
- **Special tests.**
  - **Adson's test:** Indicates occlusion of subclavian artery.
    Feel the radial pulse while abducting, extending, and
    externally rotating.

- **Ankle clonus:** May indicate UMN lesion. Quickly dorsiflex the foot while cradling the heel in your palm to relieve the load.
- **Bakody sign:** Indicates cervical radiculopathy. Patient raises his or her hand on top of the head.
- **Compression:** Indicates nerve root tension/radiculopathy. With the patient seated, press downward on top of the skull.
- **Distraction:** Indicates nerve root tension/radiculopathy. Pull upward on skull.
- **Doorbell sign:** Indicates nerve root tension/radiculopathy. Deep palpation of C5.
- **Halstead maneuver:** Neurovascular compression. In a seated patient, palpate a radial pulse, and then pull traction on the patient's arm downward while the patient extends the head backward.
- **Hoffmann's sign:** Myelopathic sign. Flick the patient's DIP joint of the long finger.
- **Jackson's compression:** Nerve compression. Patient is seated and bends the head obliquely backward; then apply downward pressure on patient's head.
- **Lhermitte's sign:** May indicate spinal canal stenosis, multiple sclerosis, cervical disk impingement, or tumor. Bend the patient's head forward.
- **Rust's sign:** Test for a severe sprain or subluxation. Patient holding the weight of his or her head in the hands or lifting the head manually when arising from lying down are positive signs.
- **Swallowing:** Indicates anterior spine/prevertebral space swelling.
• **Order appropriate radiographs.**
  - **AP:** Evaluate the lateral masses, equal separation of spinous processes, best view for vertical compression fractures, equal disk spaces.
  - **Lateral:** Each cervical vertebra, cartilaginous disk space, cervical lordotic curve, C2 neural arch, lamina, spinous process, lateral mass and articular facet.
  - **Swimmer's:** If the body of C7 not well visualized on lateral view.
  - **Odontoid:** Visualize dens.

SELECTED REFERENCES

Beyer CA, Cabanela ME, Berquist TH. Unilateral facet dislocations and fracture-dislocations of the cervical spine. J Bone Joint Surg Br 1991;73:977–981.

Dellestable F, Gaucher A. Clay shoveler's fracture. Stress fracture of the lower cervical and upper thoracic spinous processes. Rev Rheum Engl Ed 1998;65:575–582.

Foster MR. C1 fractures. Available at: http://www.emedicine.com/orthoped/topic31.htm. Accessed January 26, 2005.

Mahoney BD. Spinal Injuries. In: Tintinalli JE, Krone RL, Ruiz E, eds. Emergency Medicine: A Comprehensive Study Guide. 4th Ed. New York: McGraw Hill; 1996:1147–1153.

McCulloch PT, France J, Jones DL, et al. Helical computed tomography alone compared with plain radiographs with adjunct computed tomography to evaluate the cervical spine after high-energy trauma. J Bone Joint Surg Am 2005;87:2388–2394.

Morton RE, Khan MA, Murray-Leslie C, et al. Atlantoaxial instability in Down's syndrome: a five-year follow-up study. Arch Dis Child 1995;72:115–119.

Steel H. Anatomical and mechanical considerations of the atlanto-axial articulations. J Bone Joint Surg Am 1968;50:1481–1482.

Woodring JH, Lee C. Limitations of cervical radiography in the evaluation of acute cervical trauma. J Trauma 1993;34:32–39.

3

Thoracic and Lumbar Spine

ANATOMY

The bone anatomy of the thoracic and lumbar spine is shown in Figure 3.1. The thoracic and lumbar vertebrae (typical vertebrae) are shown in Figures 3.2 and 3.3.

Specifically, the anatomy of the thoracic and lumbar spine includes:

Body (centrum): Mass of the vertebrae; along with the disk, it supports the weight of the entire skeleton.
- **Thoracic spine:** Heart-shaped body, limited motion compared to the lumbar spine.
- **Lumbar spine:** Broad, kidney-shaped; largest movable vertebrae.

Pedicles: Form the base of the vertebral arch bilaterally.

Laminae: Extend from the pedicles, and fuse with each other at the spinous process. Laminae become thicker as the column descends.

Spinous processes: Posterior projection.
- **Thoracic spine:** Long and slender. Middle processes gain inferior slope, but as they approach the lumbar segments, they become horizontal.
- **Lumbar spine:** Short, blunt, and horizontally oriented.

Transverse processes: Arise from the lateral aspects of the vertebral arches between the pedicle and lamina.

Longitudinal ligaments (Fig. 3.4).
- **Anterior longitudinal ligament:** Runs the length of the anterior surface of the vertebral bodies and disks. Its origin is on the anterior surface of the foramen magnum to the sacrum. A hyperextension (whiplash) injury to the cervical spine implies tears in the anterior longitudinal ligament.
- **Posterior longitudinal ligament:** Runs along the posterior aspect of the vertebral body, within the vertebral canal. Its

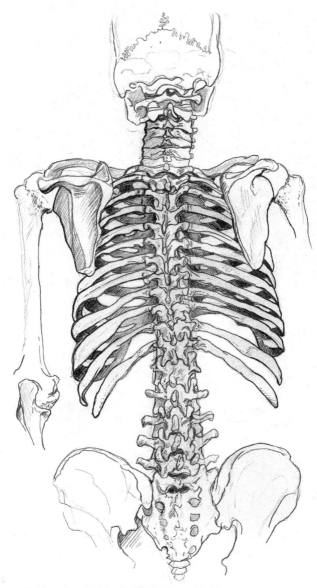

Figure 3.1 Bony anatomy of the thoracic and lumbar spine.

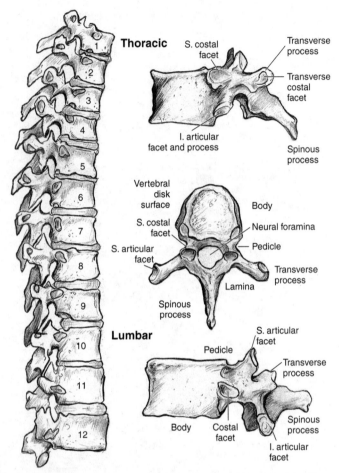

Figure 3.2 T1 to T12 (typical vertebrae), showing costal facets and demifacets. I., inferior; S., superior.

superior attachment is the occipital bone and internal aspect of the foramen magnum.

Ligamentum flavum: These accessory ligaments extend from the superior laminae at the anteroinferior border to the posterosuperior border of the inferior vertebrae.

Articular facets: Two superior and inferior facets articulate with the vertebrae above and below it. These are termed *zygapophyseal joints.*

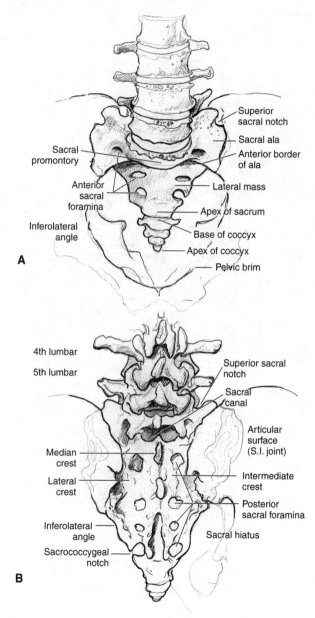

Figure 3.3 L1 to sacrum. **a:** anterior. **b:** posterior.

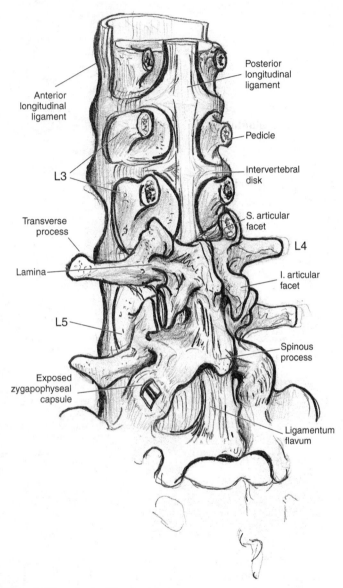

Figure 3.4 Longitudinal ligaments.

Costal facets: Articulate with ribs on the vertebral body; one or more facets according to level. The ribs also articulate with the transverse process laterally.

Vertebral canal (neuroforamina): Formed by the body (anteriorly), paired lamina (laterally), and spinous process (posteriorly); contains the spinal cord. The thoracic canal is circular, whereas the lumbar canal is more oval or triangular.

Intervertebral disk: Fibrocartilaginous plates composed of an outer **annulus fibrosis** surrounding an inner highly elastic and avascular **nucleus pulposus.** The obliquely oriented, fibrous attachments between the plates and adjacent vertebral bodies are very strong and rarely torn. Bone is more likely than disks to shear (i.e., Chance fracture through vertebral body). Disks become thicker as they descend.

Note: In this chapter, the anatomic charts have been arranged according to disk level, because the orthopaedic examination pertaining to the back is commonly oriented as such. Again, note that much of back pain pathology is related to muscular and not vertebral pathology (Fig. 3.5). Spinal surgery does lie within the realm of orthopaedic procedures, whereas muscular injury is treated with immediate rest, nonsteroidal anti-inflammatory drugs (NSAIDs), and return to exercise.

BASIC EXAMINATION

In the setting of trauma, a complete neurologic and motor examination is mandatory. This is performed while spinal precautions are maintained, and appropriate imaging should precede advanced assessment. Assessment of the nontraumatic lumbar spine can be both difficult and confusing. Observation, especially of gait and standing posture, can add a great deal of information. Patients with back pain often complain of pain in the hip and buttocks, and hip joint pain often is localized to the groin. A chronic history of back pain lends itself to lumbar vertebrae pain, however the vast majority of thoracolumbar pain is musculoskeletal in nature. Specialized tests, such as the straight-leg and well-leg raise, as well as the Patrick's test and the Gaenslen's sign, can help distinguish between lumbar disk pain and sacroiliac pain. Pain with spinal motion in the setting of infection raises the suspicion of intrathecal infection, such as meningitis, and can be reinforced by the presence of a positive Kerning's or Brudzinski's sign.

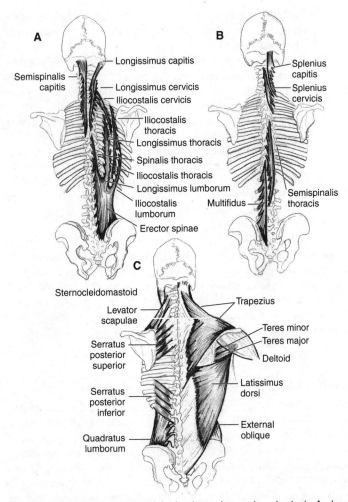

Figure 3.5 Muscular anatomy of the lumbar spine. **a:** deep intrinsic. **b:** deep intrinsic. **c:** superficial, prime movers.

In the absence of trauma to the lumbar spine, it can be taken through a full range of motion:

Flexion	60–90°
Extension	5–15°
Lateral movement	10–20°
Rotary movement	5–15°

While standing, the patient should perform forward flexion and extension at the waist. Lateral flexion and lateral rotation are apparent on palpation of spinous process separation. Note that the spine deviates to the painful side of flexion with disk herniation and root irritation. Ankylosing spondylitis leaves the entire spine rigid; therefore, these patients lack rotatory movement and have decreased expansion on deep breathing.

The approximate arrangement of function to spinal segment is:

L2: Hip flexors (iliopsoas).
L3: Knee extensors (quadriceps).
L4: Ankle dorsiflexors (tibialis anterior).
L5: Big toe extensors (extensor hallucis longus).
S1: Ankle plantar flexors (gastrocnemius and soleus).

Instruct the patient to heel walk to test L5. Have the patient toe walk or rise up and down repeatedly on the toes to test S1.

Tables 3.1 and 3.2 outline the basic muscular organization and innervation of the thoracic and lumbar spine.

Reflexes should also be examined. In the deep tendon, examine:

- **Patellar reflex:** This is the most familiar reflex and is performed by tapping the patellar tendon corresponding to the L4 nerve root.
- **Achilles reflex:** Tap the common plantar tendon (Achilles) to illicit plantar flexion corresponding to the S1 nerve root.

Also examine:

- **Superficial lumbar reflexes.**
  - **Abdominal:** Stimulate the anterior abdominal quadrant to contract that quadrant.
  - **Cremasteric:** Stimulate the inner thigh to contract the ipsilateral scrotum.
- **Anal reflex:** Contraction of the anal sphincter with palpation.

Note: Absence of any of these spinal reflexes implies an upper motor neuron (UMN) lesion.

SPECIAL TESTS
Babinski Test and Oppenheim Test

These core neurologic tests of central nervous system pathology involve running a fingernail/hammer handle up the bottom of feet (Babinski test [Fig. 3.6]) or tibial crest (Oppenheim test). The stimulus should be stiff

Table 3.1 Muscles of the Spine

Disk	Muscles	Reflex	Sensation
T12, L1, L2, L3, and L4	Iliopsoas (hip flexor)		Lateral femoral cutaneous nerve anterior thigh group
L2, L3, and L4	Quadriceps group: Quad extension	Patellar	Femoral nerve
L4	Hip extension: Tibialis anterior (lower leg dorsiflexion and eversion)	Patellar	Deep peroneal nerve medial leg, medial to tibial crest
L5	Extensor hallucis longus: Resists toe extension Gluteus medius: Hip abduction Extensor digitorum longus: Lesser toe extension	No reflex (posterior tibial is a weak and difficult reflex)	Deep peroneal
S1	Peroneus longus and brevis (plantar flexion and eversion)	Achilles	Superficial peroneal nerve lateral malleolus, plantar aspect of foot
S1 and S2	Gastrocnemius–soleus group (calf flexion)	Achilles	Tibial nerve
S1	Gluteals (prone hip extension)	Achilles	Inferior gluteal nerve
S2, S3, and S4	Bladder and intrinsic foot muscles		Anus
L3 and L4	Anterior tibialis	Patellar	Median leg and median foot
L4 and L5	Extensor hallucis longus	None	Lateral leg and dorsum of foot
L5 and S1	Peroneus longus and brevis	Achilles	Lateral foot

Table 3.2 Muscular Anatomy of the Thoracic and Lumbar Spine

Muscles	Origin	Insertion	Action
Superficial			
Trapezius	Occiput, C7 to T12 (spinous processes)	Acromion, scapular spine, lateral third of clavicle	Scapular adduction, rotation, elevation, and depression
Rhomboid major	T2 to T5 (spinous processes)	Medial scapular border	Scapular adduction
Rhomboid minor	C7 to T1 (spinous processes)	Medial scapular spine	Scapular adduction
Levator scapulae	C1 to C4 (transverse processes)	Superior, medial scapula	Scapular elevation
Serratus posterior superior	C7 to T3 (spinous processes), ligamentum nuchae, supraspinal ligament	Ribs 2–5	Elevated ribs
Serratus posterior inferior	T11 to L3 (spinous processes), supraspinous ligament	Ribs 9–12	Depresses ribs
Latissimus dorsi	T7 to T12 spinous processes, iliac crest	Intertubercular groove of humerus, in groove	Adduction and medial arm rotation
Deep			
Splenius muscles[a]	T1 to T6 (spinous processes), inferior ligamentum nuchae		Independently they laterally flex and rotate the skull. Together, they extend the neck

(continued on next page)

Table 3.2 Muscular Anatomy of the Thoracic and Lumbar Spine *(Continued)*

Muscles	Origin	Insertion	Action
Splenius capitis		Mastoid process, occiput	
Splenius cervicis		C1 to C4 (transverse processes)	
Erector spinae	Common tendon, which inserts at iliac crest, sacrum, lumbar spinous process		
Iliocostalis (lateral)	Common tendon	Iliocostalis: Angle of ribs, C4 to C6	Back extensors, release in flexion
Longissimus (intermediate)	Common tendon	Longissimus cervicis: Superior thoracic and cervical transverse processes	Back extensors, release in flexion
		Longissimus capitis: Mastoid process	
		Longissimus thoracis: Transverse processes of all thoracic vertebrae, inferior nine ribs	
Spinalis (medial)	Common tendon	Lumbar and thoracic spinous processes	Back extensors, release in flexion
Transversospinalis	Traverse distance from spinous process (SP) to transverse process (TP)		All these deep muscles stabilize the spine

Table 3.2 Muscular Anatomy of the Thoracic and Lumbar Spine *(Continued)*

Muscles	Origin	Insertion	Action
Semispinalis	SP to TP	Semispinalis cervicis and thoracis: Insert at superior spinous process Semispinalis capitis: Inserts at occiput	Combined cervical and thoracic extensors and unilateral rotators
Multifidus	SP to TP (S4 to C2)	Vertebral arches to spinous processes	Unilateral flexors and rotators of trunk, combined extensors
Rotatores	SP to TP	Deepest layer: Vertebral arches to spinous processes	Rotate superior vertebrae to opposite side
Interspinous	SP and TP	Superior vertebral SP and TP	Assistance in back extension

but not painful. A positive test is splaying and plantar flexion of the toes, with great toe extension; this result indicates the presence of a UMN lesion.

Bechterew's Test

A sitting patient is asked to extend one leg at a time and then both legs. A positive test is electrical or shooting leg pain, which indicates radiculopathy.

Bonnet's Sign

This test involves thigh adduction. A positive test is pain on stretching the piriformis, which indicates sciatica or local piriformis damage.

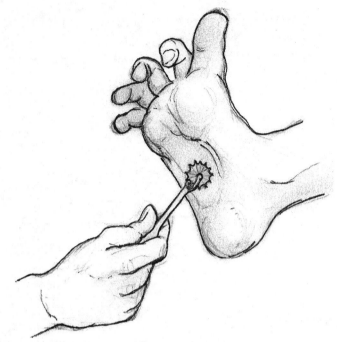

Figure 3.6 Babinski test.

Brudzinski's Sign

This chin-to-chest movement (see Fig. 3.9) provokes a flexion of the knee, thus preventing stretching of meninges in meningitis.

Gaenslen's Sign

Patient lies supine with knees to chest and then lowers one leg off the edge of the examination table, which stresses the sacroiliac joint (Fig. 3.7).

Hibbs Test

This test is used to indicate sciatica. Place the patient in a prone position with a straight leg. Maximally extend and externally rotate the leg (this internally rotates the hip and stretches the piriformis). Pain at the sacroiliac joint indicates a sacroiliac lesion, hip pain indicates hip

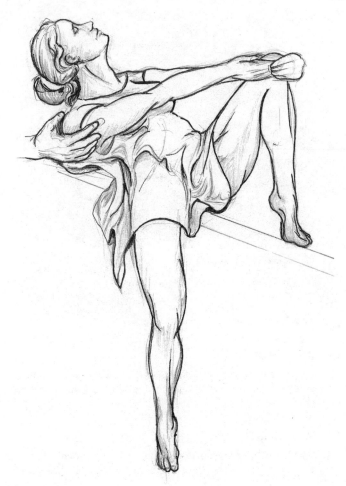

Figure 3.7 Gaenslen's sign.

lesion/sprain, and pain radiating down the back of the leg indicates piriformis entrapment of the sciatic nerve.

Hoover's Test

The Hoover's test (Fig. 3.8) is a test for malingering. Hold the heels
while the patient tries to perform a leg lift. Normally, the opposite foot
should be levered down.

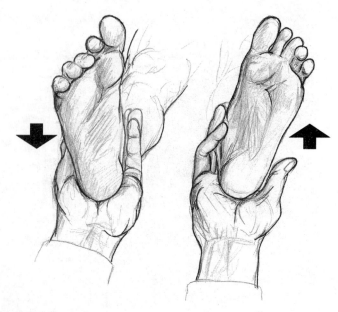

Figure 3.8 Hoover's test.

Kerning's Sign

This knee-to-chest movement stretches the spinal cord and meninges, suggesting irritation or inflammation (Fig. 3.9). A positive test is pain in the back and neck.

Lewin Supine Test

If patient is unable to perform a sit-up because of local or radiating pain, it could indicate either lumbar arthritis, spondylolisthesis, sciatica, or possibly, disk herniation.

Milgram's Test

This test involves holding bilateral leg raises. A positive test is the inability to hold for more than 30 seconds, suggesting intra-, extra-, or thecal pathology. This test stresses the iliopsoas and abdominals.

Patrick's Test

In the Patrick's test (Fig. 3.10), have a supine patient run the heel up the contralateral shin. Press at the hip and the bent knee to stress the hip and sacroiliac joint.

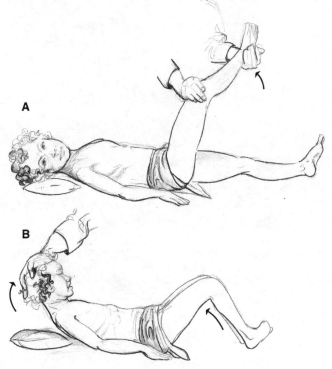

Figure 3.9 a: Kerning's sign. **b:** Brudzinski's sign.

Pelvic Rock

This test stresses the sacroiliac joint.

Straight-Leg Raise Test

The straight-leg raise (Fig. 3.11) is used to indicate that pain is probably radicular (sciatic nerve). A positive test is pain on leg raise and foot dorsiflexion.

Waddel's Signs

This is a nonorganic and psychosocial component of the examination. The presence of three of the following five signs usually is indicative of malingering:

1. Pain with light touch (out of proportion to examination).
2. Pain with axial rotation of the pelvis and axial loading of the top of the skull.

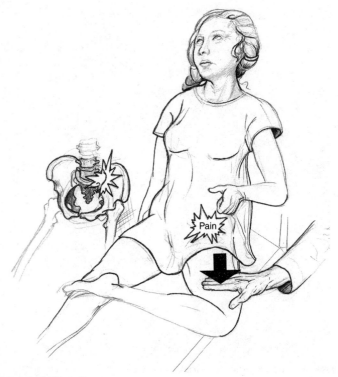

Figure 3.10 Patrick's test.

3. Strength discrepancy between sitting straight-leg and lying straight-leg raises.
4. Nonanatomic weakness or sensory (dermatomal) changes.
5. Overreaction.

Well-Leg Raise

The well-leg raise (Fig. 3.11) also indicates the presence of a space-occupying lesion (e.g., a herniated disk) if the patient has back and sciatic pain in the opposite side.

Yeoman's Test

In a prone patient, stabilize the sacroiliac joint with one hand, and lift the painful straight leg, bend the knee, and hyperextend the thigh (Fig. 3.12). A positive test indicates a sacroiliac joint origin/pathology.

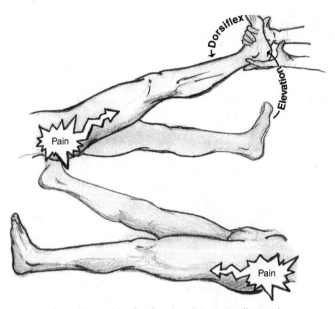

Figure 3.11 Straight-leg raise **(top)** and well-leg raise **(bottom)**.

RADIOLOGIC APPROACH TO THE THORACIC AND LUMBAR SPINE

Overview

When evaluating a patient with spinal trauma and neurologic deficits or any sudden onset of neurologic symptoms, the decision to perform magnetic resonance imaging (MRI) should be swift. Early treatment with intravenous steroids has produced considerable decreases in morbidity in cases of spinal cord contusion and hematomas, which may occur in the absence of occult fractures and need quick recognition and treatment.

Plain-film radiographs almost always are the initial choice for evaluating the spine; however, as in the case of the cervical spine, computed tomography (CT) can impart great sensitivity and specificity. Often fractures are seen to be more complex than first thought when viewed with CT. Differentiation between **compression fractures** and **burst fractures** is important (Table 3.3) and changes the clinical management. Burst fractures, by definition, are comminuted vertebral body fracture with fragments intruding into the neural canal, often requiring surgical management.

Approximately 90% of fractures in the thoracolumbar region are between segments T12 and L4, so this interval should be scrutinized in

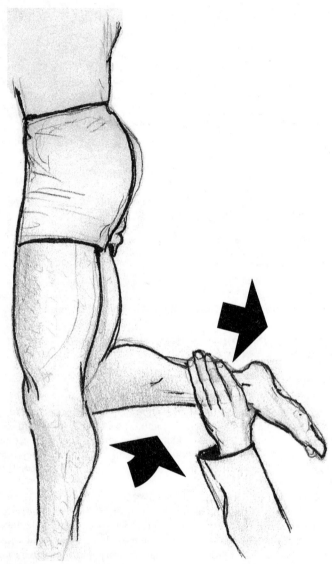

Figure 3.12 Yeoman's test.

Table 3.3 Fracture Characteristics

	Burst Fracture	**Compression Fracture**
Body height	>50% compression of body	<50% compression
Compression angle	>20°	<20°
Posterior vertebral body angle	>100°	<100°
Cortex	Disruption of cortex	No disruption

the setting of trauma and back pain. Pain is not necessary if the mechanism of injury is serious. Bending or lifting injuries often do not require radiography; the yield of positive findings in the radiograph of nontraumatic back pain is very low.

Some indications for thoracolumbar radiography are:

- **Significant trauma:** Motor-vehicle (including motorcycle) accidents involving ejection.
- **Known or suspected cervical spine injury.**
- **Altered level of consciousness or intoxication.**
- **Long fall:** >10–15 feet.
- **In elderly patients:**
  - **Known primary cancer:** Suspected metastatic disease (especially prostate, multiple myeloma).
  - **Osteoporosis or prolonged steroid use.**
  - **Significant distracting injury.**
  - **Ankylosing spondylitis, osteogenesis imperfecta, and other such conditions.**

Views

Note: Check to make sure you have the correct patient, the correct date, and the correct anatomy.

The standard thoracolumbar views to obtain are the anteroposterior (AP) (Fig. 3.13), lateral (Fig. 3.14), and spot views of the L5 to S1 interspace. Add oblique views (Fig. 3.15) if pedicle, laminar, or facet fractures or dislocations are suspected.

The important radiographic observations in all views are:

- **Height of the vertebral bodies:** Is it maintained?
- **Normal alignment of the spine.**
- **Normal distances between the vertebrae at the intervertebral disk.**

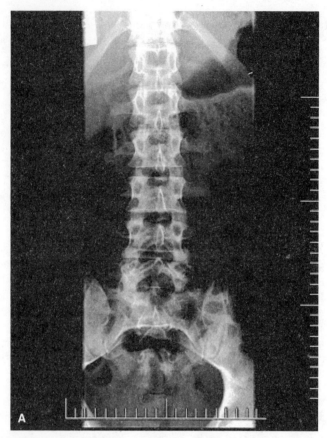

Figure 3.13 a: Anteroposterior radiograph of the lumbar spine.
(continued on next page)

- **Spaces, facet joints, and spinous processes.**
- **Presence of parallel surfaces of the joints and vertebral end plates.**
- **Midline spinous processes and lateral transverse processes:** Can they be followed?

To develop a better eye for abnormal radiographs and comfort with radiographs in general, it helps to identify normal anatomic landmarks verbally (on rounds) or mentally. As in all of orthopaedics, comparisons with contralateral or adjacent structures (in this case, vertebrae) can reveal a great deal. Although significant gradual change in vertebral

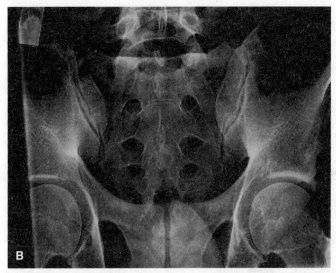

Figure 3.13 *(continued)* **b:** Anteroposterior radiograph of the lumbar spine (sacrum).

structure occurs as the column descends toward the pelvis, any abrupt change or focal finding is suspicious.

Anteroposterior View

The adequate AP radiograph contains the majority of the thoracic or lumbar spine, especially the thoracolumbar junction. Penetration should be sufficient to depict vertebral bodies through the overlying cardiac shadow. Vertebral bodies should not be rotated, and spinous processes should be centered.

Identify the major structures on the AP view: transverse and spinous processes, pedicles, bodies, and intervertebral disk space. The **BACKPAINS** mnemonic has been used in some texts and is helpful for identifying some key landmarks.

Bone
Alignment
Cartilage
Kyphosis
Paraspinal and psoas lines
Apophyseal joints
Interpedicular and interspinous distances
Neuroforamina
Scoliosis

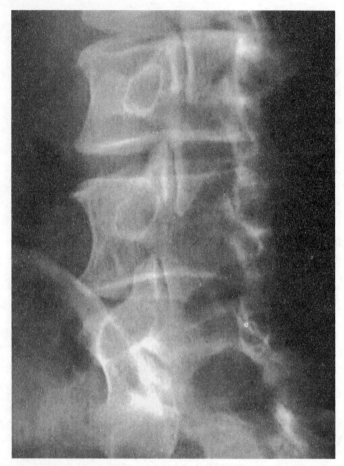

Figure 3.14 Lateral radiograph of the lumbar spine.

Loss of the psoas line has good sensitivity for picking up vertebral fractures and often shows widening of the paraspinal line. The interpedicular and interspinous distances also are disrupted with fracture.

Lateral View

An adequate lateral radiograph shows good depiction of pertinent vertebrae and no rotation (Fig. 3.14). The three columns of the spine can be scrutinized on the lateral view and the distances compared. Superior and inferior end plates should be clearly seen and undisrupted.

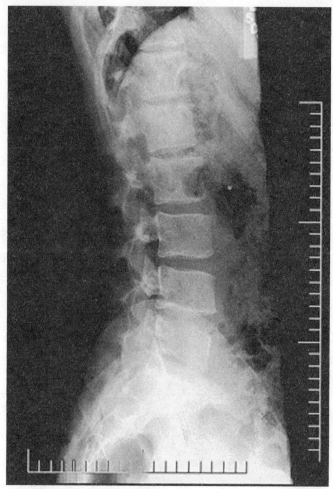

Figure 3.15 Oblique radiograph of the lumbar spine.

The height and width of the vertebral bodies should be approximately equal, not pie-shaped. Slight kyphosis in the thoracic spine and a gentle lumbar lordosis are normal.

Oblique View

The purpose of the oblique view is to better depict the intervertebral foramina and zygapophyseal joints (Fig. 3.15). The now-familiar "scotty dog" should be outlined at each level and never be "wearing his collar"

(Fig. 3.16). The collar is an indication of spondylolysis (chronic) at the pars articulation or facet fracture (acute).

SELECTED FRACTURES OF THE THORACIC AND LUMBAR SPINE

Burst Fractures

The lumbar burst fracture (Fig. 3.17) is again related to axial loading; however, it most commonly results from a significant fall in which the patient lands on the heels and force is translated upward. Usually,

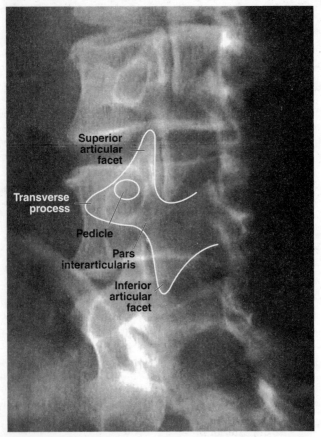

Figure 3.16 Oblique radiograph of the lumbar spine ("scotty dog"). A "collar" or break in the neck of the dog corresponds to a fracture in the region of the pars articularis, which is specific for spondylolysis.

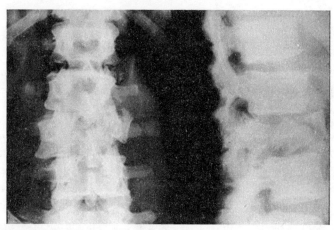

Figure 3.17 Radiograph of a burst fracture.

these are stable fractures unless the patient has greater than 50% of vertebral body height collapse and greater than 25–35° of kyphosis. The mechanism of injury and the forces placed on the annulus fibrosis and vertebral body leave a large central posterosuperior fragment. Steroids may be indicated if neurologic deficits are noted or strongly suspected. Examination can include evaluation for the presence of an ileus. Treatment is conservative for stable fractures, and a variety of operative decompressions and fusions are indicated for unstable fractures.

Anterolateral Compression Fractures (Chance Fractures)

This fracture pattern is most common in the setting of a rapid deceleration motor-vehicle accident, usually with the occupant wearing a lap belt only. Because of the relative strength of the ligamentous attachments of the disks to the vertebrae, a horizontal fracture occurs across the vertebral body. This represents a failure of all three columns of the spine, most often L2 and L3. In this flexion/distraction-type injury pattern, approximately half the patients have ligamentous rupture (interspinous and ligamentum flavum); however, neurologic compromise is relatively rare. Make a diagnosis on the basis of lateral radiographs, but an AP view is necessary to rule out fracture of posterior processes. Also, if needed, use a CT. Scrutinize the spinous process, lamina, pedicles, and portion of the vertebral body. Nonoperative cases have less than 15° of kyphosis on a lateral radiograph.

Spondylolysis and Spondylolisthesis

These terms often are lumped together and are interrelated, affecting the same spinal structure (the pedicle and spinal facet).

Spondylolysis

In spondylolysis, there is a nonfused pedicle, which is attached to the vertebral body by soft tissue structures only. This is thought to be a nonunion stress fracture during childhood development. If spondylolysis is present, it makes the vertebrae below it susceptible to a facet dislocation or spondylolisthesis.

Spondylolisthesis

In spondylolisthesis, the superior articular facet of the inferior vertebrae "slips" posteriorly to the inferior articular facet of the superior vertebrae. Symptoms are proportional to the degree of slip and the amount of tension that is placed on the spinal cord, roots, and disk. Pain is not a necessary symptom of spondylolisthesis. Diagnosis is via plain-film radiography, CT, or MRI. Treatment often is nonsurgical and similar to nontraumatic back pain, for which strengthening exercises are indicated. Significant refractory pain or high-degree slips may be treated surgically. Traumatic spondylolisthesis is not uncommon in motor vehicle accidents.

SELECTED DISORDERS OF THE THORACIC AND LUMBAR SPINE

Ankylosing Spondylitis

This disorder belongs to the larger family of the seronegative spondyloarthropathies. A T-cell and macrophagic synovitis and release of cytokines (e.g., tumor necrosis factor-α and tumor growth factor-β), with the resultant destruction and remodeling of bone, accounts for the pathophysiology of the disease. This disorder has a clear genetic component, supported by the findings that patients most often are negative for rheumatoid factor and positive for HLA B27. The peak incidence is 15–30 years of age. Common targets are the sacroiliac joint, vertebrae, aorta, and aortic valves. Ankylosing spondylitis often affects the sacroiliac joints first and eventually, the spine, which becomes lordotic. A "bamboo spine" on a radiograph, showing fusion (ankylosis) of vertebrae, is characteristic. Restriction of chest expansion can be a fatal complication of this disease. Treatment is NSAIDs and physical therapy.

Multiple Myeloma

Multiple myeloma is a malignancy of plasma cells and the leading primary cause of malignancy in bone (the second leading cause is osteogenic sarcoma). Metastatic spread is the overall leading cause of bone cancer. Cellular proliferation is monoclonal in origin and is manifested by a characteristic spike on serum protein electrophoresis. This is a disease of the elderly, with peak incidence among people in their 70s. Bone pain (most often back pain) is the most common presenting symptom. Pathological fractures are common in advanced disease, as are fatigue and weakness. Other symptoms include increased susceptibility to infection (decreased normal immunoglobulin production) and pain and swelling in the ribs, skull, sternum, or other sites. Anemia is a prominent component of disease, and rouleaux formation may be seen on the peripheral smear. Bence Jones proteins (immunoglobulin light chains) are detected in the urine, as are hypercalcemia in the blood and an elevated erythrocyte sedimentation rate. The textbook characterization of radiographic findings is "punched out" lytic bone lesions in the skull, sternum, and long bones. Chemotherapy is the first-line treatment, although currently, no consensus exists regarding specific drug regimens.

Intervertebral Disk Disease

With aging, the intervertebral disk loses its resiliency, and damage to the fibrocartilaginous outer disk can occur. This results in extrusion of the nucleus pulposus gelatinous center, most often posterolaterally. Cord or nerve root compression can result in radiculopathy and pain that shoots down the leg from the hip. The condition can be reproduced by the well-leg and the straight-leg raise.

Postmenopausal Osteoporosis

In the normal premenopausal female, estrogen down-regulates osteoclast-activating factor (interleukin-1) from active osteoblasts. In the absence of normal estrogen levels, osteopenia results from a relative increase in bone breakdown. Pathological findings include vertebral body stress fractures (the most common presenting symptom), radial styloid fracture (Colles' fracture), overall loss of height, and a kyphotic cervical spine (dowager's hump).

Nonmodifiable risk factors include:

Gender: Women (68%) are affected more than men.
Age: Risk increases with age.
Body size: Small, thin women are at greater risk.
Ethnicity: Asians and Caucasians have the highest risk.
Family history: A history of fractures carries a greater risk.

Modifiable risk factors include low estrogen (in women), low testosterone (in men), anorexia, low calcium and vitamin D intake, cigarettes, inactivity, alcohol use, and certain medications.

Urinary concentrations of osteocalcin and pyridinium collagen cross-links is one test to measure skeletal collagen loss, which is a marker of bone loss (resorption). The other main test is the bone mineral density (BMD) test, which uses various radiologic methods to assess bone density. The reason for obtaining a BMD test is to assess the risk of fracture. The BMD test is a very good predictor, and it should be obtained for the following patient populations:

1. Postmenopausal patients who are not on hormone replacement therapy (HRT) but who are concerned about osteoporosis prevention and would consider HRT, bisphosphonates, or selective estrogen-receptor modulators if the test results suggest low BMD.
2. Maternal history of hip fracture, smoking, height greater than 5'7", or weight less than 125 pounds.
3. Patients on medications associated with bone loss (antiestrogens).
4. A history of conditions associated with low bone mass (e.g., hyperthyroidism, posttransplantation, malabsorption, hyperparathyroidism, or alcoholism).
5. Increased osteocalcin and pyridinium urinary collagen cross-links.
6. Previous known or suspected fragility fracture.

A DEXA Scan (Dual-energy x-ray absorptrometry) is the preferred test currently for determining bone mineral density. Two main scores are obtained from this information, the T score and the Z score. The T score is the number of standard deviations above or below the young adult mean. The Z score is the number of standard deviations the patient's bone density is above or below the values expected for that patient's age. T scores of ± 1 are normal, -1 to -2 is generally considered osteopenic, and > -2.5 is osteoporotic.

The U.S. Preventive Services Task Force recommends that osteoporosis screening be started in women 65 years and older. Dual-energy x-ray absorptiometry, the test of choice, yields a T and Z score. Women who are considered to be at high risk because of low weight or estrogen deficiency should be screened at 60 years of age.

Cauda Equina/Conus Medullaris Syndrome

If the inferior fibers of the spinal cord (Fig. 3.18) are compressed or the blood supply is compromised at the lumbar level, one of these two syndromes may result, depending on the level:

- **Cauda equina:** Symptoms usually are gradual in onset and unilateral and consist of weakness to unilateral paraplegia, absent reflexes,

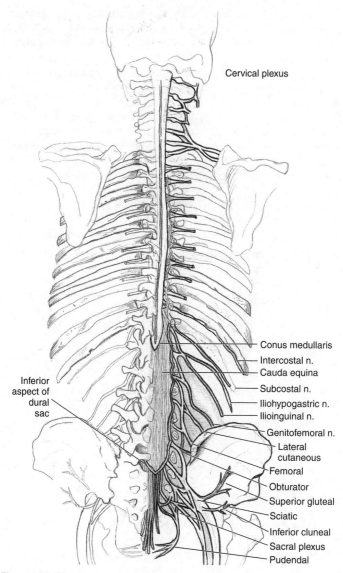

Cervical plexus

Conus medullaris

Intercostal n.

Cauda equina

Subcostal n.

Iliohypogastric n.

Ilioinguinal n.

Genitofemoral n.

Lateral cutaneous

Femoral

Obturator

Superior gluteal

Sciatic

Inferior cluneal

Sacral plexus

Pudendal

Inferior aspect of dural sac

Figure 3.18 Distribution of spinal nerve, roots and dural sac. n., nerve.

and paresthesia in an asymmetric saddle distribution to the anus, with the perineum sometimes extending to dermatomes of the lower extremity. In contrast to conus medullaris syndrome, greater lower motor neuron (LMN) symptoms, such as severe radicular pain, occasional impotence, and urinary retention, also may be present.

- **Conus medullaris:** Because of the higher level of this lesion (distal spinal cord), UMN symptoms are more frequent and prominent. Onset is faster than in cauda equina, and symptoms are more likely to be bilateral and symmetric in the saddle distribution. Symmetric, hyperreflexive paresis and fasciculations are present, but ankle reflexes are absent. Impotence and urinary retention have an earlier onset and are more severe than in cauda equina syndrome.

Some common causes of both syndromes include lumbar stenosis, spinal trauma, herniated disk, neoplasm (astrocytoma, neurofibroma, and meningioma), infection/abscess, and idiopathic or iatrogenic causes (e.g., spinal anesthesia). Treatment options are both medical (steroids) and surgical (decompression).

Quick Look • Lumbar Spine

Note: If the patient is taking cervical spine precautions, evaluate the patient while he or she is in the cervical collar, or remove the collar while the head is immobilized by a second caregiver.

- **Inspect** the skin and posture, looking for gross deformity.
- **Palpate** down the length of the spinous process, note crepitus, swelling, or step-offs.

If no trauma:

- **Move back through range of motion.**
  - **Flexion:** Forward bend (observe alignment of the spine), 60–90°.
  - **Hyperextension:** Lean back, 5–15°.
  - **Lateral bending:** Side to side, 10–20°.
  - **Axial rotation:** Rotation at hips, 5–15°.
- **Observe gait.**
  - **Normal:** Smooth and fluid, with some overlap.
  - **Heel walk to test L5.**
  - **Toe walk.**
- **Reflex testing** if neurologic deficits, lumbar stenosis, or UMN/LMN disorder is suspected or if the patient is preoperative or postoperative.

- **Patellar (L4), Achilles (S1).**
- **Abdominal, cremasteric, bulbocavernosus, anal.**
  - **Absent:** Neuropathy, LMN lesion.
  - **Hyperactive:** UMN lesion.
- **Special tests.**
  - **Babinski's and Oppenheim's tests:** UMN lesion.
  - **Bechterew's test:** A sitting patient is asked to extend one leg at a time and then both legs; radiculopathy.
  - **Bonnet's sign:** Thigh adduction, sciatica.
  - **Brudzinski's sign:** Chin to chest; suggests irritation or inflammation.
  - **Gaenslen's sign:** Hang one leg off the examination table; stresses the sacroiliac joint.
  - **Hibbs's test:** Sciatica.
  - **Hoover's test:** Malingering.
  - **Kerning's sign:** Knee to chest; suggests irritation or inflammation.
  - **Lewin's supine test:** Cannot perform a sit-up because of local or radiating pain; lumbar arthritis, spondylolisthesis, sciatica, or possibly, disk herniation.
  - **Milgram's test:** Rules out intrathecal pathology; stresses iliopsoas and abdominals.
  - **Patrick's test:** Run one heel up the contralateral shin, and apply pressure at the knee; stresses the hip and sacroiliac joint.
  - **Pelvic rock test:** Stresses the sacroiliac joint.
  - **Straight-leg raise:** Space-occupying lesion/sciatica.
  - **Well-leg raise:** Space-occupying lesion/sciatica.
  - **Yeoman's test:** Lift the painful straight leg; bend the knee, and hyperextend the thigh; sacroiliac joint pathology.
- **Order appropriate films.**
  - **AP:** Evaluate bone, alignment, cartilage, kyphosis, paraspinal and psoas lines, apophyseal joints, interpedicular and interspinous distances, neuroforamina, and scoliosis.
  - **Lateral:** Scrutinize the distances of the three columns. Evaluate superior and inferior end plates for symmetry. The height and width of the vertebral bodies should be roughly equal, not pie-shaped.
  - **Oblique:** Visualize the intervertebral foramina and zygapophyseal joints. Check "scotty dog."

SELECTED REFERENCES

Anderson PA, Rivara FP, Maier RV, et al. The epidemiology of seatbelt-associated injuries. J Trauma 1991;31:60–67.

Bennett DL, Ohashi K, El-Khoury GY. Spondyloarthropathies: ankylosing spondylitis and psoriatic arthritis, Radiol Clin North Am 2004;42:121–134.

Canale S. Circulation of spinal cord. Campbell's Operative Orthopaedics 1998;9:2683.

Esses SI, Botsford DJ, Kostuik JP. Evaluation of surgical treatment for burst fractures. Spine 1990;15:667–673.

Goljan EJ. STARS Pathology. Philadelphia: WB Saunders, 1998.

International Myeloma Foundation. Initial or Frontline Therapy for Multiple Myeloma. Available at: http://myeloma.org/main.jsp?tab_id=2&type=article&id=743. Accessed December 15, 2005.

Krompinger WJ, et al. Conservative treatment of fractures of the thoracic and lumbar spine. Orthop Clin 1986;17:161–170.

Mau W, Zeidler H, Mau R, et al. Clinical features and prognosis of patients with possible ankylosing spondylitis: results of a 10-year follow-up. J Rheumatol 1988;15:1109–1114.

Miller PD, Siris ES, Barrett-Connor E, et al. Prediction of fracture risk in postmenopausal white women with peripheral bone densitometry: evidence from the National Osteoporosis Risk Assessment. Bone Miner Res 2002;17:2222–2230.

Seybold EA, Sweeney CA, Fredrickson BE, et al. Functional outcome of low lumbar burst fractures. A multicenter review of operative and nonoperative treatment of L3-L5. Spine 1999;24:2154–2161.

U.S. Preventive Services Task Force. Screening for Osteoporosis in Postmenopausal Women: Recommendations and Rationale. September 2002. Agency for Healthcare Research and Quality, Rockville, MD. http://www.ahrq.gov/clinic/3rduspstf/osteoporosis/osteorr.htm. Accessed December 20, 2005.

4

Shoulder

ANATOMY

The bony, muscular, and vascular anatomy of the shoulder girdle and the upper arm are shown in Figure 4.1.

Bones of the Shoulder Girdle

Clavicle

Also known as the "collar bone," the clavicle is a roughly S-shaped bone forming the anterior portion of the shoulder girdle that articulates with the sternum and scapula. It is frequently fractured.

Scapula

Acromion: Anterolateral extension of the scapula that articulates with the clavicle. The anterior origin of the deltoid and anterior insertion for the trapezius, this forms part of the acromioclavicular (AC) joint, which is commonly disrupted following trauma.

Coracoid: Anterior process of the scapula and origin for the short head of the biceps and coracobrachialis.

Glenoid: Shallow, cup-shaped articulation with the humeral head that is surrounded by cartilaginous labrum. It is the site of Bankart and superior labrum anterior–posterior (SLAP) lesions.

Infraglenoid tubercle: Origin of the long head of the triceps.

Scapular spine: Posterior origin of the deltoid, and posterior insertion of the trapezius.

Supraglenoid tubercle: Origin of the long head of the biceps.

Humerus

Anatomic neck: Site of the glenohumeral (GH) capsule attachment.

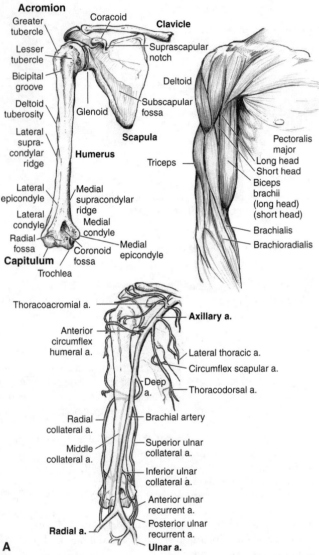

Figure 4.1 Bony, muscular, and vascular anatomy of the shoulder girdle and upper arm. **a:** Anterior view.

(continued on next page)

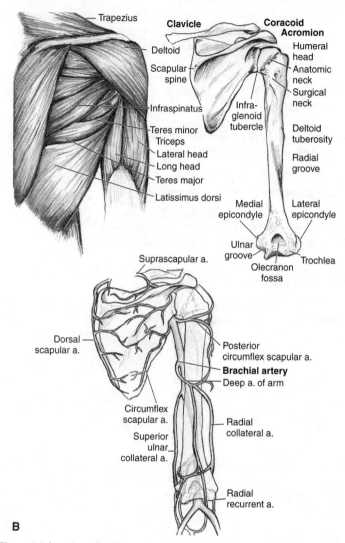

Figure 4.1 *(continued)* **b:** Posterior view. a., artery.

Deltoid tuberosity: Insertion point for the deltoid muscle.

Head: Smooth and semispherical; articulates with the glenoid fossa.

Intertubercular (bicipital) groove: Grooved depression in the humeral neck and head that transmits the long head of the biceps tendon. The transverse humeral ligament is superior to the tendon that restrains it. Disruption of the ligament causes pain and popping with use.

Surgical neck: Narrowing distal to the greater and lesser tubercles; the common site for fractures that could involve both the axillary nerve and the posterior circumflex artery.

Tubercles.

- **Greater tubercle:** Attachment for the supraspinatus, infraspinatus, and teres minor muscles.
- **Lesser tubercle:** Attachment for the subscapularis muscle.

Articulations of the Shoulder Girdle

Glenohumeral: Plane joint.
Sternoclavicular: Gliding (double-plane) joint.
Acromioclavicular: Multiaxial ball-and-socket joint.

Muscles of the Shoulder

The shoulder, a complex and dynamic joint, involves the motion of bones and muscles in many planes (Tables 4.1 and 4.2). Sensory distribution via cervical and thoracic nerve roots uses this following pattern (Fig. 4.2):

Lateral arm	C5
Medial arm	T1
Axilla	T2
Axilla to nipple	T3
Nipple	T4

Note: The deltoid patch is pure C5.

Figure 4.3 shows the axillary and brachial arteries. Figure 4.4 shows shoulder cutaneous sensation.

BASIC EXAMINATION

One should note that many muscles of the upper back are prime movers of the shoulder and should be factored into the differential diagnosis of shoulder problems. Although a history of trauma factors into assessment of the shoulder joint complex to a great extent, specialized testing can be used effectively to distinguish between the various muscles and bony processes of the shoulder. Pain on palpation, especially of the AC joint and bicipital groove, can be telling.

Table 4.1 Muscles of the Shoulder

Muscle	Origin	Insertion	Action
Deltoid	Lateral clavicle, acromion, scapular spine	Deltoid tuberosity	**AB**duction, **AD**duction, extension, medial rotation
Supraspinatus[a]	Scapula, supraspinous fossa	Greater tubercle of humerus, superior	Abducts arm
Infraspinatus[a]	Scapula, infra-spinous fossa	Greater tubercle of humerus, middle	Lateral arm rotation
Teres minor[a]	Upper portion of dorsal lateral scapula	Greater tubercle of humerus, inferior	Lateral arm rotation
Subscapularis[a]	Ventral scapula, subscapular fossa	Lesser tubercle of humerus	Medial arm rotation
Teres major	Dorsal inferior scapula	Intertuber-cular groove of humerus, medial	**AD**duction and medial arm rotation
Latissimus dorsi	T7 to T12 spin-ous processes, iliac crest	Intertuber-cular groove of humerus, in groove	**AD**duction and medial arm rotation
Pectoralis major	Medial clavicle, sternal margin	Intertuber-cular groove of humerus, lateral	**AD**duction and medial arm rotation
Pectoralis minor	Ribs 2–7	Coracoid process	Stabilizes scapula

[a]Member of supraspinatus, infraspinatus, teres minor, and subscapularis (SITS) group of muscles comprising the musculotendinous rotator cuff.

Table 4.2 Innervation of the Shoulder Muscles

	Specific Muscle	**Nerve (Root)**
Abductors		
Prime mover	Middle deltoid	Axillary nerve (C5 and C6)
	Supraspinatus	Subscapular nerve (C5 and C6)
Secondary mover	Anterior and posterior deltoid Serratus anterior (via scapula)	
Adductors		
Prime mover	Pectoralis major	Medial and lateral anterior thoracic nerve (C5, C6, C7, C8, and T1)
	Latissimus dorsi	Thoracodorsal nerve (C6, C7, and C8)
Secondary mover	Teres major	
Shoulder flexors		
Prime mover	Anterior deltoid Coracobrachialis	Axillary nerve (C5) Musculocutaneous nerve (C5 and C6)
Secondary mover	Pectoralis major Biceps brachii Anterior deltoid	
Shoulder extensors		
Prime mover	Latissimus dorsi	Thoracodorsal nerve (C6, C7, and C8)
	Teres major	Lower subscapular nerve (C5 and C6)
	Posterior deltoid	Axillary nerve (C5 and C6)
Secondary mover	Teres minor Triceps (long head) Anterior deltoid	
External rotation		
Prime mover	Infraspinatus	Suprascapular nerve (C5 and C6)
	Teres minor	Axillary nerve (C5)
Secondary mover	Posterior deltoid	

(continued on next page)

Table 4.2 Innervation of the Shoulder Muscles *(Continued)*

	Specific Muscle	Nerve (Root)
Internal rotation		
Prime mover	Subscapular	Upper and lower subscapular nerve (C5 and C6)
	Pectoralis major	Medial and lateral anterior thoracic nerve (C5, C6, C7, C8, and T1)
	Latissimus dorsi	Thoracodorsal nerve (C6, C7, and C8)
	Teres major	Lower subscapular nerve (C5 and C6)
Secondary mover	Anterior deltoid	
Scapular elevation		
Prime mover	Trapezius Levator scapulae	Cranial nerve XI (C3 and C4)
Secondary mover	Rhomboids	
Scapular retraction		
Prime mover	Rhomboid major	Dorsal scapular nerve (C5)
	Rhomboid minor	Dorsal scapular nerve (C5)
Secondary mover	Trapezius	
Scapular protraction		
Prime mover	Serratus anterior	Long thoracic nerve (C5, C6, and C7)

Specific examination tips include:

- Passive extension allows palpation of the supraspinatus, infraspinatus, teres minor, and subscapularis (SITS) muscles.
- Palpate inferior to the cuff muscles for bursae (shoulder girdle), then palpate the muscles of the shoulder girdle, sternocleidomastoid, pectoralis major, biceps, trapezius, and rhomboids (Fig. 4.5).
- Move the patient through range of motion (ROM) (Fig. 4.6), and use the tests detailed in this chapter to help localize the lesion (Table 4.3):

Abduction	180°
Adduction	50°

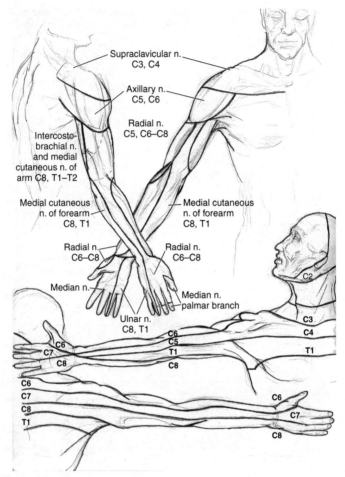

Figure 4.2 Motion correlates with spinal level. n., nerve.

Flexion	180°
Extension	50°
Internal rotation	55°
External rotation	45°

Palpation

It is necessary to palpate the suprasternal notch, sternoclavicular joint, clavicle, coracoid, AC joint, acromion, greater tuberosity of humerus,

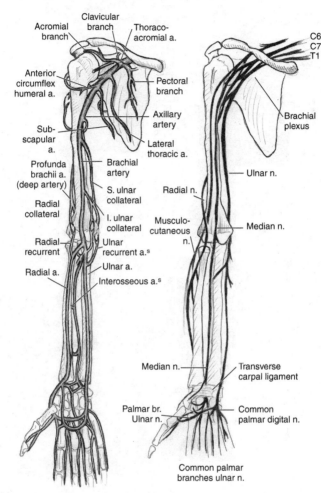

Figure 4.3 Axillary and brachial arteries. a., artery; I., inferior; n., nerve; S., superior.

bicipital groove, lesser tuberosity of the humerus, and scapula. Palpate the soft tissues surrounding the following structures:

- Rotator cuff.
- Subacromial and subdeltoid bursa.
- Axilla.
- Muscles of the shoulder girdle.

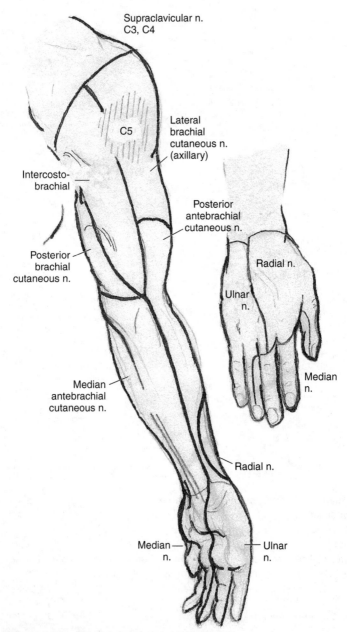

Figure 4.4 Shoulder cutaneous sensation. n., nerve.

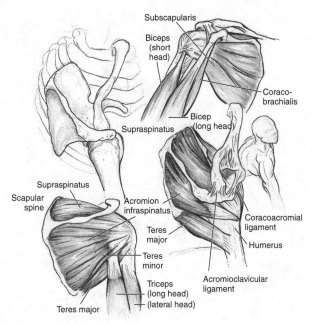

Figure 4.5 Musculotendinous rotator cuff.

SPECIAL TESTS

Anterior Slide Test

The anterior slide test (Fig. 4.7) is a test of joint capsule instability. Place upward pressure on the humerus at the elbow. A positive test is anterior/superior translation of the GH joint.

Apprehension Test

The apprehension test (Fig. 4.8) is a test for joint instability/dislocation. Abduct and externally rotate a 90° flexed arm, stressing the anterior labrum/capsule (most common site of dislocation [90% of cases]), and apply a torque in the posterior direction to stress the posterior labrum/capsule. A positive test is pain and instability in the anterior aspect (or in the posterior aspect when the reverse torque is applied).

Crank Test

This is a test for a glenoid labral tear. Elevate the shoulder 160° internally, and externally rotate the humerus while applying an axial load. A positive test is shoulder pain and crepitus (grinding or popping).

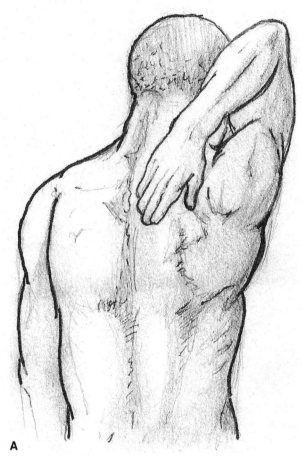

A

Figure 4.6 Range-of-motion. **a:** Flexion.
(continued on next page)

Cross-Arm Test

The cross-arm test (Fig. 4.9) is a test of AC arthrosis. Rotate the humerus in 90° forward flexion across the chest. A positive test is pain at the AC joint.

Drop Arm Test

This is a test for deltoid insufficiency/rotator cuff tear. Fully abduct the arm, and then slowly lower it. A positive test is the sudden drop of the arm to the side. Pain or weakness indicates "painful arc syndrome" (bur-

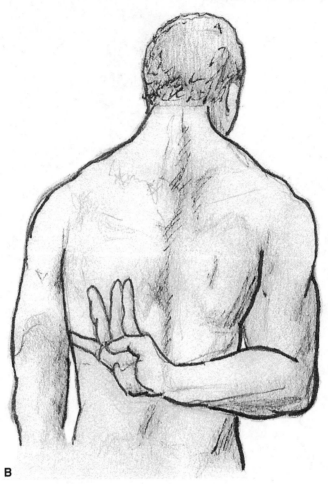

Figure 4.6 *(continued)* **b:** Internal rotation.
(continued on next page)

sitis, rotator cuff strain, tendonitis, or impingement). Inability to maintain a 90° abducted position against gravity (less than +3/5 muscle strength) indicates severe injury (grade 3 cuff tear).

Dugas Test

If the hand of the affected side is placed on the opposite shoulder, the elbow cannot touch the chest. A positive test is the inability to complete the test, which indicates anterior GH dislocation.

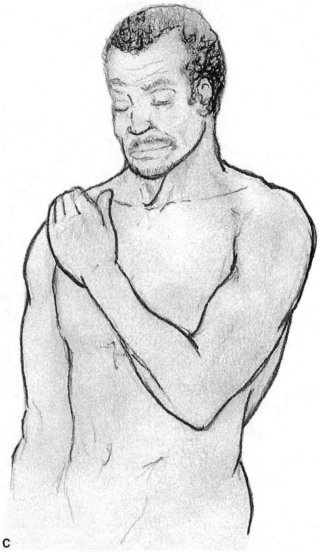

C

Figure 4.6 *(continued)* **c:** Adduction.

Table 4.3 Tests Used in Examination of Shoulder

Muscle/Process	Test
Supraspinatus	Abduction, Hawkins, O'Brien
Subscapularis	Internal rotation, lift-off, Napoleon
Infraspinatus	External rotation
Teres minor	Somewhat with extension
Deltoid	Abduction, flexion, drop arm, atrophy
Latissimus	Pull down, adduction
Acromioclavicular joint	Impingement, pain on palpation

Elevated Arm Stress Test

Also known as the East test, this is a test for thoracic outlet syndrome. In a sitting patient with the arms abducted 90° from the thorax and the elbows flexed 90°, instruct the patient to open and close the hands for 3 minutes. Patients with thoracic outlet syndrome are unable to perform this for 3 minutes because of reproduction of symptoms. Carpal tunnel syndrome produces dysesthesias in the finger but no pain in the shoulder or arm.

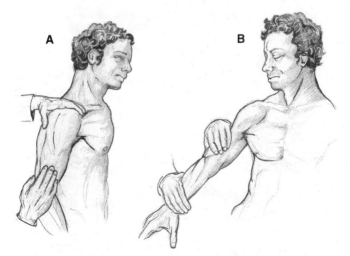

Figure 4.7 Anterior slide (**a**) and O'Brien (**b**) tests.

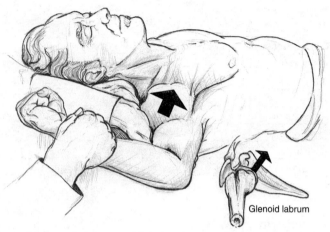

Glenoid labrum

Figure 4.8 Apprehension test, showing that anterior force on the humeral head precipitates a sensation of dislocation at the glenoid labrum.

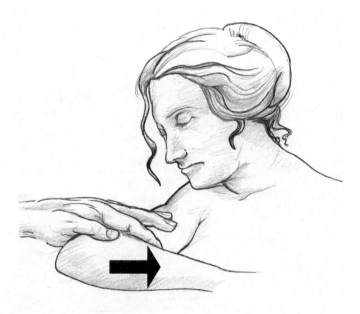

Figure 4.9 Cross-arm test.

Hawkin's Test

The Hawkin's test (Fig. 4.10) is a test of AC joint impingement and supraspinatus tendon weakness/tear. This is the same test as the impingement sign except that the thumb is pronated, thus involving more supraspinatus action.

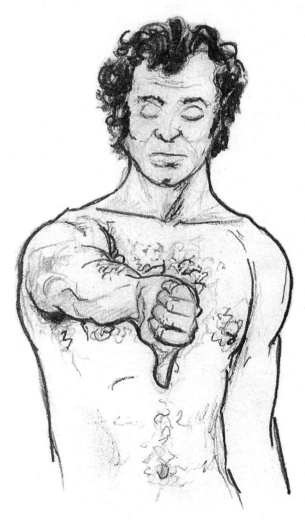

Figure 4.10 Hawkin's test.

Impingement Sign

The impingement sign (Fig. 4.11) is a test of AC joint impingement of the supraspinatus tendon. The test involves passive forward flexion of greater than 90°. A positive test is AC joint pain, which indicates impingement.

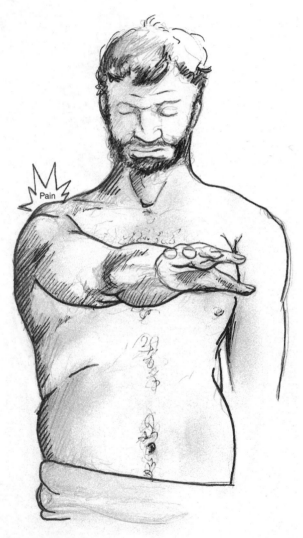

Figure 4.11 Impingement sign.

Jobe's Test (Empty Beer Can Test)

Also known as the empty beer can test, the Jobe's test is a test for the relative isolation of the supraspinatus. The patient rotates the upper extremity with the thumbs pointing to the floor. Resistance is applied with the arms in 30° of forward flexion and 90° of abduction. A positive test is unilateral weakness, which suggests disruption of the supraspinatus tendon.

Lift-off Test

In the lift-off test (Fig. 4.12), the patient reaches behind the back for the scapula (indicates anterior capsule ROM). Ability to lift the hand off the back indicates an intact subscapularis.

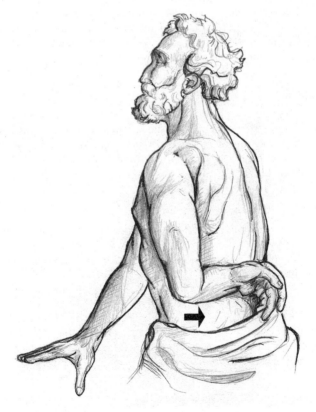

Figure 4.12 Lift-off test.

Load Shift Test

This is a test of posterior cruciate ligament instability. Laterally abduct the humerus to 90° while applying axial force, and move into 90° of forward flexion. Pain, apprehension, posterior instability, subluxation, or dislocation implies posterior capsule insufficiency.

Napoleon's Test

With the hands flat on the stomach in a "chicken" position, the ability to bring the elbows past the frontal plane indicates an intact subscapularis.

O'Brien Test

The O'Brien test (Fig. 4.7) is a test for a SLAP lesion (glenoid labral and biceps tendon tear). With the shoulder in 90° of forward flexion and 30° of adduction, the patient resists forward flexion while the thumbs are pointed downward, rotates to full supination, and resists forward flexion again. A positive test is a painful thumb when pointed downward and a shoulder click with supination.

Scapular Winging Test

In the scapular winging test (Fig. 4.13), positive flaring of the scapula indicates paresis or paralysis of the serratus anterior muscle. Subtle posterolateral winging indicates paresis or paralysis of the trapezius muscle. These injuries result from a spinal accessory lesion or a severed long thoracic nerve.

Shoulder Hiking Test

A patient with a weak or injured rotator cuff (especially a supraspinatus tendon), decreased GH mobility (frozen shoulder), or significant osteoarthritis compensates by hiking up the shoulder, using trapezius and scapular action.

Sulcus Sign

The sulcus sign (Fig. 4.14) is a test of ligamentous laxity. Pull the humerus in an inferior direction, and look for an inferior subluxation/dislocation gap (sulcus sign).

Yergason's and Speed's Tests

These are tests for bicipital groove stability/pathology. The Yergason test (Fig. 4.15a), which involves external rotation with a flexed elbow,

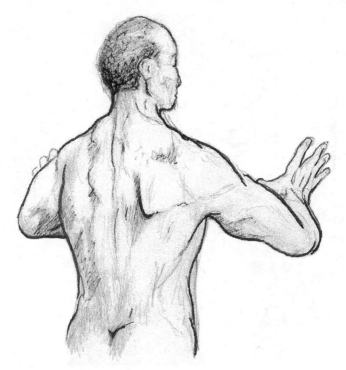

Figure 4.13 Scapular winging test.

tests the stability of the biceps tendon in the groove. The Speed's test (Fig. 4.15b) is the same but adds forward elevation. A positive result is pain.

RADIOLOGIC APPROACH TO THE SHOULDER
Overview

There is little doubt that the shoulder is a difficult and complex structure to evaluate. Adequate radiographic evaluation requires good technique and a knowledge of anatomy. As usual, errors in reading shoulder radiographs can be reduced by following a systematic approach and identifying anatomic landmarks either verbally or mentally. Pertinent structures and areas of concern include the clavicle, AC joint, greater and lesser tuberosities, GH joint, humeral neck, and scapular body and neck. The margins of the shoulder radiograph contain the chest wall and ribs; these are worth viewing because identification of a fractured humerus should not cause the neglect of

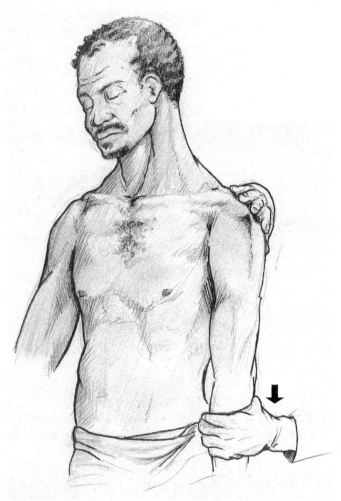

Figure 4.14 Sulcus sign.

fractured ribs or a pneumothorax. Cortices and trabeculae should be scrutinized for fractures, especially in the elderly and in chronic steroid users. The hot light often is useful for examining the AC joint in overpenetrated films. A suspicion of avascular necrosis should be present in patients with sickle cell disease and in chronic steroid users. Although unicameral (most common) and aneurysmal bone cysts are rare, the proximal humerus is a common site for these cysts.

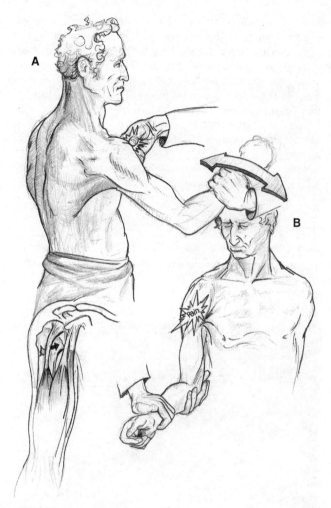

Figure 4.15 a: Yergason test. **b:** Speed's test. The figure shows the biceps tendon "popping" out of the bicipital groove.

Views

Three views are standard:

1. Anteroposterior (AP) in internal and external rotation.
2. Lateral (scapular Y).
3. Axillary.

A posterior oblique (Grashey) view is useful to obtain a clear depiction of the GH joint. Computed tomography may be necessary to determine the extent of fractures involving the glenoid labrum. Stress views with the patient holding a weight also may be helpful to evaluate AC joint injuries but rarely affect management. Posterior dislocations (infrequent) often are missed because of failure to seek them out as a result of the mechanism of injury and use of the proper views (axillary and scapular Y). If examination raises the suspicion of scapular or clavicular fractures, then additional views should be requested and evaluated.

Note: Check to make sure you have the correct patient, the correct date, and the correct anatomy.

Anteroposterior View

A good AP radiograph of the shoulder (Fig. 4.16) often entails two films with the humerus in internal and external rotation to obtain

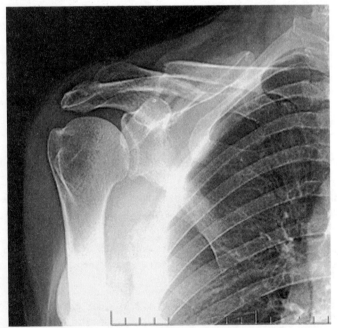

Figure 4.16 Anteroposterior radiograph of shoulder.

frontal and lateral views of the greater tuberosity. In internal rotation, the lesser tuberosity overlies the GH.

The AP view should be evaluated for:

- Fractures, especially at the surgical neck, greater and lesser tuberosities, and glenoid labrum (Bankart lesion).
- AC joint space (3–5 mm is normal; >1 cm indicates AC separation).
- Tendon locations for calcification (overuse injury).

Lateral (Scapular Y) View

With the scapular Y view (Fig. 4.17), a Y-intersection of lines can be drawn from the coracoid, acromion, and body of the scapula. The intersection of these lines is the glenoid fossa, where the humeral head should be seen. If the intersection is anterior to this point, the humeral head is dislocated. This view helps identify fractures of the humerus and scapula but is most useful for dislocations; whereas the axillary view requires abduction of the patient's arm, the scapular Y does not and is ideal following painful trauma. This also provides a direct frontal view of the glenoid. Scapular fractures can be minimally displaced and may only be evident as a thin, white line of overlapping bone.

Axillary View

The axillary view involves abduction of the arm and is painful to patients with fractures of the glenoid labrum humeral head and acromion as well as those with anterior and posterior dislocations. An adequate radiograph provides good visualization of the glenoid rim and GH joint.

Posterior Oblique View

In the patient who is suspected of having a posterior dislocation or degenerative joint, an oblique view provides a lateral view of the GH joint and joint space.

SELECTED FRACTURES AND DISLOCATIONS OF THE SHOULDER

Shoulder Dislocations

Although relocating a dislocated shoulder probably falls outside the realm of basic orthopaedic examination maneuvers, an overview of the procedures for relocation should be mentioned. Note that these procedures do pose a risk of further and significant shoulder damage as well as fracture of the humeral head.

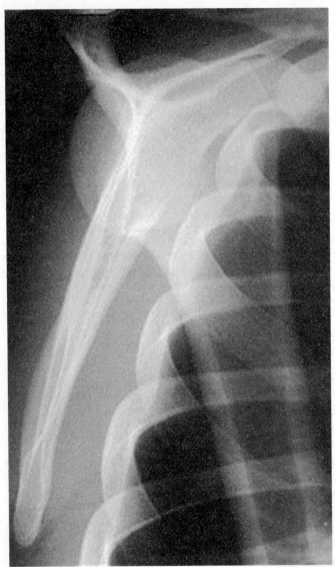

Figure 4.17 Scapular Y radiograph.

Types

Initial evaluation of a suspected dislocation begins with identifying the external **appearance of a dislocated shoulder:**

- **Anterior dislocation** (90%; most common type): Usually occurs following a traumatic fall on an outstretched, abducted, externally rotated arm. This type is sometimes characterized by the mnemonic **TUBS:**
    Traumatic injury
    Unilateral injury
    Bankart labral tear or Hill-Sachs GH fractures
    Surgical management, which is often necessary

Other characteristics include:

- A much more prominent acromion.
- Possible presence of a positive sulcus sign without the application of traction.
- Significant reduction in the ROM of the joint.
- Usually, holding of the arm adducted and in external rotation, with painful internal rotation.

- **Posterior dislocation:** Often seen as a double shoulder shadow on a scapular Y view. It is sometimes characterized by the mnemonic **AMBR:**
    Atraumatic
    Multidirectional instability present prior
    Bilateral or history of bilateral instability
    Rehabilitation, which often is indicated for treatment

Other characteristics include:

- Arm held by the patient in internal rotation, with the arm often resting on the abdomen.
- Painful external rotation.

Treatment

Rapid management often aids in the reduction of these injuries—before muscular spasm is well set in. Sedation and relaxation often is sufficient to reduce the shoulder, possibly with the addition of a small amount of traction applied to the arm. The two most popular means of reducing the dislocated shoulder are the sedation traction/countertraction technique and the Kocher maneuver:

- **Sedation (Stimson) technique** (Fig. 4.18): Provide adequate sedation and pain management using midazolam (Versed) and morphine. A small, 5- or 10-pound weight often is attached to the distal arm in a prone patient.
- **Traction/countertraction** (Fig. 4.19): Place traction at the wrist, parallel to the body, in a seated or supine patient while a sheet or towel is wrapped around patient's trunk under the axilla. Pull countertraction posteriorly across the chest, possibly upward at 30°.
- **Kocher maneuver** (Figs. 4.20, 4.21, and 4.22): In a sitting or supine patient, adduct and flex the arm while externally rotating it. Slowly internally rotate in a flexed arm to relocate. This maneuver should be done gently and early to avoid complications. Significant muscle spasm makes this very difficult.

Note: Pre- and postprocedural neurovascular checks are mandatory, as are postreduction films.

Superior Labrum Anterior–Posterior and Bankart Lesions

Bankart lesions involve detachment of the anterior labral cartilage from the glenoid rim and are more common than SLAP lesions. They usually are related to trauma and are complications of shoulder dis-

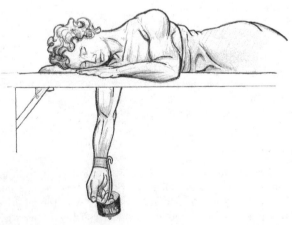

Figure 4.18 Stimson technique.

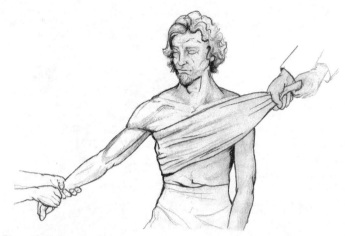

Figure 4.19 Traction/countertraction.

locations. The SLAP lesions are tears of the labral cartilage in the GH joint and also may involve the origin and anchor of the biceps brachii tendon. The GH joint is responsible for the majority of shoulder motion and stability in addition to absorption of compressive and directional forces by the labrum. One theory of this pathology is that posterior capsular tightness leads to stretching and tearing of the anterior capsule by a levering action of the humeral head on the posterior labrum, leading to joint laxity and instability.

These injuries are classified as types I to VII:

- **Type I:** Stable and only involve small amounts of fraying or degeneration.
- **Type II** (most common): Complete tears of the superior labrum, where it attaches to the glenoid.
- **Types III and IV:** More extensive and are only attached on each end of a superior tear, giving it a bucket-handle appearance.
- **Type IV:** Involves the biceps tendon.
- **Type V** (anteroinferior Bankart lesion): Full separation of the biceps tendon.
- **Type VI:** Separation of the biceps tendon in addition to an unstable labral flap tear.
- **Type VII:** Combined superior labral and biceps tendon separation, which extends into the middle GH ligament.

When seeking treatment, patients complain of clicking in the shoulder or even locking. Bankart lesions often are related to trauma and

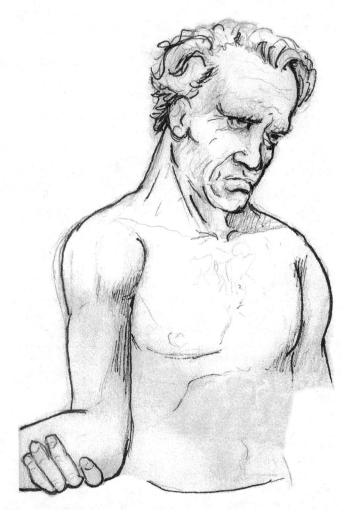

Figure 4.20 Kocher maneuver: Arm flexion, adduction, external rotation.

forceful anterior dislocation. Many times, these lesions are diagnosed after findings of shoulder instability, which lead to arthroscopy (although most orthopaedists suspect a Bankart or SLAP lesion going into the surgery). Results of the anterior slide, O'Brien, crank, and apprehension tests are good physical examination findings, and noncontrast magnetic resonance imaging (MRI) and T_1-weighted magnetic resonance arthrography are useful for diagnosis. Treatment options are

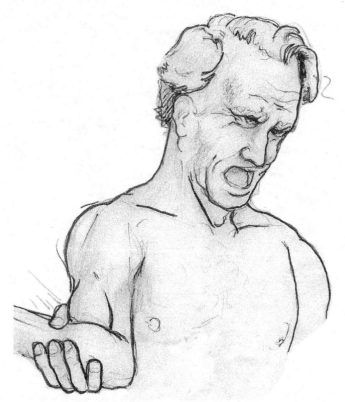

Figure 4.21 Kocher maneuver: Elevation with external rotation.

numerous and, although different, usually involve the following elements: débridement of tissue, repair of the biceps anchor, and repair of the tear. Repair of the biceps anchor can be accomplished arthroscopically by placing titanium screws, absorbable and nonabsorbable tacks, and suture anchors. There is active debate concerning the superiority of open versus arthroscopic repairs of these lesions.

Hill-Sachs Fracture

A Hill-Sachs fracture is essentially an indentation or a depressed fracture of the humeral head. Internal rotation or axillary views are preferred for visualization. Hill-Sachs fracture as well as SLAP and Bankart lesions do not necessarily imply recurrent dislocation, but they commonly occur in this setting.

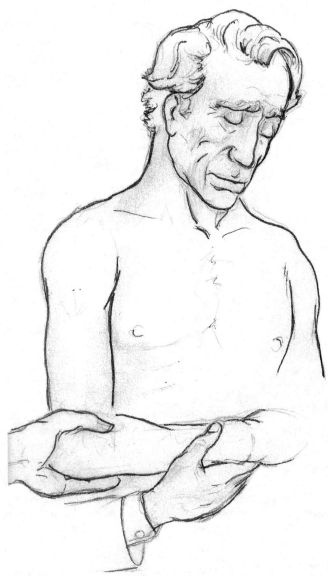

Figure 4.22 Kocher maneuver: Internal rotation.

Rotator Cuff Injury

The shoulder is a dynamic joint capable of a wide ROM. Multiple anatomic structures are responsible for maintaining the integrity and stability of the shoulder joint, including the joint capsule, labral cartilage, and musculotendinous rotator cuff. The SITS muscles (supraspinatus, infraspinatus, teres minor, subscapularis) comprise the familiar rotator cuff. The humeral head and glenoid fossa share almost perfect congruence and, therefore, create a tight fit. They articulate over a rather small surface area, however, and would create potential instability were it not for the cuff and labral extension of the cavity. Rotator cuff injuries almost always are caused by repetitive stress microtrauma that then culminates in a tear of one or more of the rotator muscles, especially in susceptible populations (the elderly) who have compromised microvascular supply and decreased tensile strength of their tendons. The anterior circumflex humeral artery, the acromial branch of the thoracoacromial artery, as well as the suprascapular and posterior humeral circumflex arteries supply the rotator cuff muscles and surrounding structures. Subacromial impingement, such as that resulting from subacromial bursitis, is a common factor in the degenerative forces on the upper cuff. In most cases, the supraspinatus tendon gives way. Throwing athletes as well as shoulder-intensive laborers are the usual victims of rotator cuff disease because of their muscle stress loads. The peak incidence for injury occurs in those in the fifties to seventies, however, and leans toward a female predominance.

The preferred tests for physical diagnosis include the lift-off, impingement sign, Hawkin's, and drop arm. Pain and weakness can be isolated by moving the shoulder through its respective ROMs. Although MRI and even ultrasound can be helpful in supporting the diagnosis, such imaging should, as with most orthopaedic pathologies, support the physical examination. Treatment is largely surgical and involves open arthroscopy and open repair of torn tendons and, often, reattachment of the tendon of the long head of the biceps to the humerus, which can be torn or ruptured. Arthroscopic débridement also is a procedure that has had satisfactory outcomes in a number of patients.

Acromioclavicular Joint Impingement/Injury

The AC joint is most often susceptible to dislocation and subluxation via a downward force applied at the tip of the shoulder. These injuries are often graded from I to VI:

- **Grade I:** Only a partial tear of the AC ligament; presents with pain on palpation.

- **Grades II and III:** A full tear (grade III also includes a torn capsule as well as the ligament).
- **Grade IV:** Posterior displacement of the clavicle through the fascia surrounding the trapezius muscle.
- **Grade V:** The clavicle is significantly superior to the acromion (by 300%), with severe inferior displacement of the GH joint.
- **Grade VI:** Clavicle pushed inferior to the coracoid process.

The diagnosis is established most precisely by radiography, but it should be readily apparent on physical examination and be suspected via the history of the mechanism of injury. A stressed AP view is performed, with the patient holding a 15- to 20-pound weight that provokes an increased distance between the acromion and the clavicle greater than 1 cm (normal <5 mm) (Fig. 4.23). Lower-grade injuries can be treated using immobilization with a sling and swath, followed by ice and anti-inflammatory medications, whereas high-grade injuries are managed surgically.

SELECTED DISORDERS OF THE SHOULDER
Thoracic Outlet Syndrome

One of the neurovascular impingement disorders, thoracic outlet syndrome is uncommon and usually related to compression via the sca-

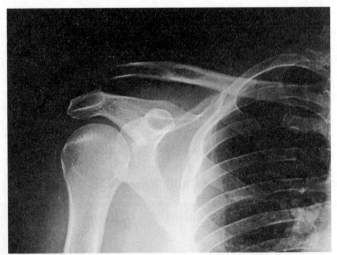

Figure 4.23 Radiograph indicating acromioclavicular joint separation (note >1 cm separation of clavicle and acromion).

lene triangle (anterior and middle scalene muscles and upper margin of the first rib). Less frequently, the presence of a cervical rib extended C7 transverse process or congenital anatomic malformations can cause a compression of the nerve root. Trauma and repetitive-use injuries are other causes of thoracic outlet syndrome and predispose musicians (who need to maintain extension/abduction for long periods). The compression of, usually, the lower two roots of the brachial plexus (C8 and T1) accounts for the neurologic sequelae associated with this disorder. Symptoms include pain, numbness, tingling, and even muscular atrophy. Symptoms often are unilateral in the distribution of the ulnar or median nerve. Thoracic outlet syndrome is a heterogeneous classification that encompasses a number of etiologies and treatment options, depending on the cause of the impingement.

Subacromial Bursitis

Painful abduction of the arm can be a sign of inflammation of this bursa. The etiology may be varied; causes include rotator cuff injury, overuse, and degenerative tendonitis. In fact, the inflammation of the subacromial bursa is believed to be one of the primary instigators of subscapularis impingement, which later results in stress and tears of the supraspinatus tendon.

Frozen Shoulder

This condition results from the accumulation of scar tissue in the shoulder joint capsule. In its primary form, frozen shoulder is idiopathic and has no identifiable etiology, whereas in its secondary form, it is attributable to various injuries or shoulder surgery. It is characterized by a slow onset and resolution and, typically, has three stages: painful, adhesive, and recovery (also known as freezing, frozen, and thawed).

Similar to rotator cuff injuries in its presentation, a history of previous surgeries or trauma is key. Radiographs usually are not helpful and show few degenerative changes. Although MRI is normal, this modality can rule out rotator cuff injury. Laboratory assays for rheumatologic and inflammatory changes are not positive. The diagnosis is established clinically by showing unilateral decreased passive and active ROM on physical examination in all planes of motion. Treatment is conservative and usually returns patient to near-normal shoulder function. Nonsteroidal anti-inflammatory drugs for inflammation as well as analgesia and opiates for pain are commonly prescribed, as are oral or injectable corticosteroids. Specific ROM exercises are instructed, and physical therapy can help mobilize the joint. Manipulation under anesthesia and arthroscopic capsule release are reserved for refractory cases.

Quick Look • Shoulder

Inspect the skin, looking for features such as gross deformity, guarding, and bruising.

Palpate the soft tissues surrounding the rotator cuff and the subacromial and subdeltoid bursae. Also palpate the bony suprasternal notch, sternoclavicular joint, clavicle, coracoid, AC joint, acromion, greater tuberosity of humerus, bicipital groove, lesser tuberosity of humerus, and scapula.

Move the shoulder through ROM.

- **Abduction:** 180°.
- **Adduction:** 50°.
- **Flexion:** 180°.
- **Extension:** 50°.
- **Internal rotation:** 55°.
- **External rotation:** 45°.

Reflex testing if neurologic deficits, cervical stenosis, or upper motor neuron (UMN)/lower motor neuron (LMN) disorder is suspected or if the patient is preoperative or postoperative.

- **Biceps (C5), brachioradialis (C6), triceps (C7).**
  - **Absent:** Neuropathy, LMN lesion.
  - **Hyperactive:** UMN lesion.

Evaluate muscles using **special tests** to isolate the disorder.

- **Anterior slide test:** Joint capsule instability. Place upward pressure on the humerus at the elbow.
- **Apprehension test:** Test for joint instability/dislocation Abduct and externally rotate a 90° flexed arm, stressing the anterior labrum/capsule. Apply torque in the posterior direction to stress the posterior labrum/capsule.
- **Crank test:** Glenoid labral tear. Rotate the humerus in 90° forward flexion across the chest.
- **Cross-arm test:** AC arthrosis. Laterally abduct the humerus to 90° while applying axial force, then move into 90° forward flexion.
- **Drop arm test:** Deltoid insufficiency. Fully abduct the arm, and then slowly lower it.
- **Dugas test:** Anterior GH dislocation. The hand of the affected side is placed on the opposite shoulder; the elbow cannot touch the chest.
- **Elevated arm stress test (East test):** Thoracic outlet syndrome. In a sitting patient with the arms abducted 90°

from the thorax and the elbows flexed 90°, instruct the patient to open and close the hands for 3 minutes.

- **Hawkin's test:** AC joint impingement of supraspinatus tendon. Passive forward flexion of greater than 90° means that the thumb is pronated.
- **Impingement sign:** AC joint impingement of supraspinatus tendon (passive forward flexion > 90°).
- **Jobe test:** Relative isolation of the supraspinatus tendon. The patient rotates the upper extremity with the thumbs pointing to the floor, and resistance is applied with the arms in 30° of forward flexion and 90° of abduction.
- **Lift-off test:** Indicates intact subscapularis. The patient reaches behind the back for the scapula and attempts to lift the hand off the back.
- **Load shift test:** Posterior cruciate ligament instability. Laterally abduct the humerus to 90° while applying axial force, and then move into 90° of forward flexion.
- **O'Brien test:** AP lesion (glenoid labral and biceps tendon tear). Put the shoulder in 90° of forward flexion and 30° of adduction. The patient resists forward flexion while the thumb is pointed downward. Rotate to full supination; patient resists forward flexion again.
- **Scapular winging test:** Paresis/paralysis of serratus anterior.
- **Shoulder hiking test:** Weak or injured rotator cuff.
- **Speed's test:** Bicipital groove stability/pathology. Same as the Yergason test but with the addition of forward elevation.
- **Sulcus sign:** Ligamentous laxity. Pull the humerus in the inferior direction, and look for an inferior subluxation/dislocation gap.
- **Yergason test:** Bicipital groove stability/pathology. External rotation with flexed elbow.

Order appropriate films.
- **AP:** Internal/external rotation if possible. Evaluate for:
  - Fractures, especially at the surgical neck, greater/lesser tuberosities, and glenoid labrum (Bankart lesion).
  - AC joint space (3–5 mm is normal, >1 cm indicates AC separation).
  - Evaluation of tendon locations for calcification (overuse injury).
- **Lateral (scapular Y):** Intersection of lines from the coracoid, acromion, and body of the scapula, where the humeral head should be seen. Anterior to this point, the humerus is

dislocated. This view helps identify fractures of the humerus and scapula but is most useful for dislocations. It also provides a direct frontal view of the glenoid.

- **Axillary:** Good visualization of the glenoid rim and GH joint.
- **Posterior oblique:** Lateral view of the GH joint in suspected posterior dislocation or degenerative joint.

SELECTED REFERENCES

Bankart AB. The pathology and treatment of recurrent dislocation of the shoulder. Br J Surg 1938;26:23–29.

Browning DG, Desai MM. Rotator cuff injuries and treatment. Prim Care 2004;31:807–829.

Cuomo F. Diagnosis, classification and management of the stiff shoulder. In: Iannotti JP, Williams GR Jr, eds: Disorders of the Shoulder: Diagnosis and Management. Philadelphia: Lippincott Williams & Wilkins, 1999:397–417.

Eskola A, Santavirta S, Viljakka S, et al. The results of operative resection of the lateral end of the clavicle. J Bone Joint Surg Am 1997; 79:633–634.

Harwood M, Smith CT. Superior labrum, anterior–posterior lesions and biceps injuries: diagnostic and treatment considerations. Primary Care: Clinics in Office Practice 2004;31:831–855.

Henry MH, Liu SH, Loffredo AJ. Arthroscopic management of the acromioclavicular joint disorder: a review. CORR 1995;316:276–283.

Information from your family doctor. Adhesive capsulitis. Am Fam Physician 2003;67:1323–1324.

Mehta S, Gimbel JA, Soslowsky LJ. Etiologic and pathogenetic factors for rotator cuff tendinopathy. Clin Sports Med 2003;22:791–812.

Melillo AS, Savoie FH III, Field LD. Massive rotator cuff tears: debridement versus repair. Orthop Clin North Am 1997;28:117–124.

Nuber GW, Bowen MK. Arthroscopic treatment of acromioclavicular joint injuries and results. Clin Sports Med 2003;22:301–317.

Oates SD, Daley RA. Thoracic outlet syndrome. Hand Clin 1996;12: 705–718.

Rawes ML, Dias JJ. Long-term results of conservative treatment for acromioclavicular dislocation. J Bone Joint Surg Br 1996;78:410–412.

Sandor R. Adhesive capsulitis: optimal treatment of "frozen shoulder." Physician Sports Med 2000;28. Available at http://www.physsports med.com/issues/2000/09/sandor.htm. Accessed December 27, 2006.

Taylor DC, Arciero RA. Pathologic changes associated with shoulder dislocations. Arthroscopic and physical examination findings in first-time, traumatic anterior dislocations. Am J Sports Med 1997;25: 306–311.

5

Elbow and Forearm

The bony upper extremity includes the elbow and forearm. Figure 5.1a shows the anterior structures of the forearm, and Figure 5.1b shows the posterior structures of the forearm.

ANATOMY

The elbow is a complex joint consisting of three articulations. Two ginglymus-type joints at the humeroradial and humeroulnar joints permit flexion/extension, and a pivot-type joint at the radial head permits pronation/supination.

Distal Humerus

Radial groove: Transmits the radial nerve closely approximated to the profunda brachial artery and is an area of danger in midshaft humerus fractures; injury results in wrist drop. Very few humerus fractures, however, result in permanent nerve damage.

Trochlea (Latin, "pulley"): The groove between the two margins of the spool-shaped pulley; articulates with the ulna through flexion/extension.

Capitulum (Latin, "little head"): Articulates with the radial head.

Olecranon fossa: Receives the olecranon on the dorsal humerus just superior to the trochlea.

Coronoid fossa: Complementary to the ulnar coronoid process.

Radial fossa: Counterpart to the radial head.

Medial epicondyle: Medial extension of the trochlea. Injury to the medial epicondyle can injure the ulnar nerve.

Lateral epicondyle: Projection of the capitulum.

Ulna

Trochlear notch: Complementary to the trochlea of the humerus.

Radial notch: Accommodates the medial radial head.

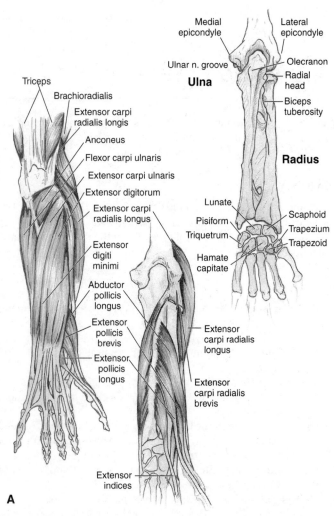

Figure 5.1 Bony upper extremity. **a:** Dorsal structures of the forearm.
(continued on next page)

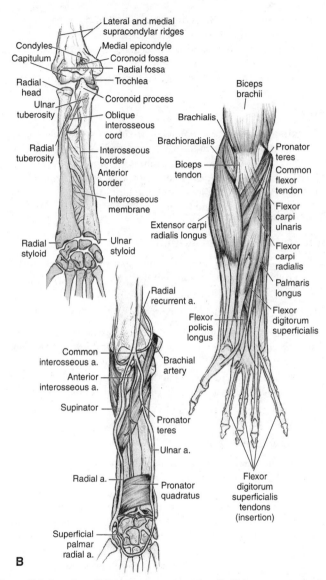

Figure 5.1 *(continued)* Bony upper extremity. **b:** Volar structures of the forearm. a., artery; n., nerve.

Olecranon: Spoon-shaped, proximal end of the ulna; the elbow serves as the site of triceps insertion.

Ulnar head: In contrast to the designation of the radial head proximally, the ulnar head is distal from the elbow, articulating with the radius and the distal radioulnar joint.

Radius

Proximal head: The radial head articulates and rotates with the capitulum of the humerus. Nursemaids' elbow involves subluxation of this joint in the annular ligament.

Radial tuberosity: Attachment for the biceps brachii.

Radial styloid: The site of the brachioradialis tendon and palpable within the anatomic "snuff box."

Muscular Anatomy and Motion

Tables 5.1 and 5.2 outline the basic muscular organization, function, and innervation involved with the elbow joint.

Vascular Anatomy and Neuroanatomy

The vascular anatomy and neuroanatomy of the upper extremity (Fig. 5.2) are relatively simple and worth remembering. The brachial plexus is a separate issue and is much more complex; however, it is not as essential to the nonorthopaedist. The key here is to note that multiple peripheral nerves are involved in a shoulder injury and that a brachial plexus injury is then suspected.

BASIC EXAMINATION

The assessment of the elbow presents a differential diagnosis that is a mixed bag of musculoskeletal and medical pathologies. The complexity of this joint cannot be overstated—but it often is underestimated. The patient history is as important as the visual and physical examination. Differentiation of medical from structural problems can be accomplished using answers to questions such as age, sex, activity, and onset of symptoms (Table 5.3). Special testing can provide strong support for nerve entrapment (cubital tunnel), cervical spinal pathology (reflex testing), and trauma/overuse (tennis elbow).

Visual Examination

The normal position of the elbow is valgus (5° males and 10–15° females). This often is described as the carrying angle.

Table 5.1	Muscles of the Elbow	
Muscle	**Origin**	**Insertion**
Upper arm		
Biceps brachii	Long head: supraglenoid tubercle Short head: coracoid	Radial tuberosity, bicipital aponeurosis
Triceps	Long head: infraglenoid tubercle Lateral head: dorsal humerus; superior to radial groove Medial head: dorsal humerus; inferior to radial groove	Olecranon
Brachialis	Distal, volar humerus	Coronoid, ulnar tuberosity
Coracobrachialis	Coracoid process	Middle, medial humerus
Anconeus	Lateral epicondyle	Olecranon, dorsal ulna
Lower arm		
Pronator teres	Medial epicondyle, coronoid process	Volar, proximal radius
Flexor carpi radialis	Medial epicondyle	Second metacarpal base
Palmaris longus	Medial epicondyle	Flexor retinaculum, palmar aponeurosis
Flexor carpi ulnaris	Medial epicondyle Olecranon and dorsal ulna	Hook of hamate, pisiform, fifth metacarpal
Flexor digitorum superficialis	Medial epicondyle, coronoid process, ulnar collateral ligament Volar radius	Middle phalanges 2–5
Deep forearm flexors		
Flexor digitorum profundus	Medial and anterior ulna	Base of phalanges 2–5
Flexor pollicis longus	Anterior radius and interosseus membrane	Base of thumb

(continued on next page)

Table 5.1 Muscles of the Elbow *(Continued)*

Muscle	Origin	Insertion
Pronator quadratus	Distal anterior ulna	Distal anterior radius
Forearm extensors		
Brachioradialis	Lateral supracondylar humerus	Lateral, distal radius
Extensor carpi radialis longus	Lateral supracondylar humerus	Base of fifth metacarpal
Extensor carpi radialis brevis	Lateral epicondyle	Base of third metacarpal
Extensor digitorum	Lateral epicondyle	Extensor expansion at digits 2–5
Extensor digiti minimi	Lateral epicondyle	Extensor expansion at fifth digit
Extensor carpi ulnaris	Lateral epicondyle, posterior ulna	Base of fifth metacarpal

Table 5.2 Muscular Motion of the Elbow

Action	Muscle	Nerve (Root)
Flexion		
Primary	Brachialis	Musculocutaneous nerve (C5 and C6)
	Biceps	Musculocutaneous nerve (C5 and C6)
Secondary	Brachioradialis Supinator	
Extension		
Primary	Triceps	Radial nerve (C7)
Secondary	Anconeus	
Supination		
Primary	Biceps	Musculocutaneous nerve (C5 and C6)
	Supinator	Radial nerve (C6)
Secondary	Brachioradialis	
Pronation		
Primary	Pronator teres	Median nerve (C6)
	Pronator quadratus	Anterior interosseus portion of median nerve (C8 and T1)
Secondary	Flexor carpi radialis	

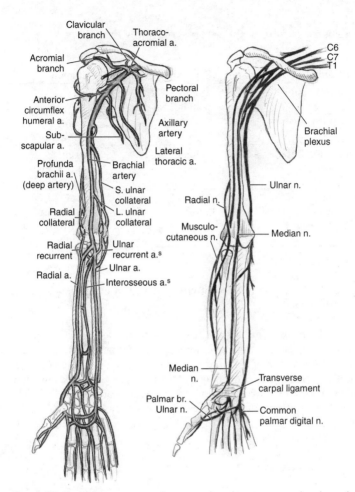

Figure 5.2 Vascular anatomy of upper extremity. a., artery; br., branch; L., lateral; n., nerve; S., superior.

Deviations from the normal angle include:

- **Cubitus varus:** In this deformity, the forearm deviates laterally from the normal elbow angle. Also called a gunstock deformity, it often is secondary to a pediatric supracondylar elbow fracture resulting in malunion or growth restriction of the medial epiphysis.
- **Cubitus valgus:** In this deformity, the forearm deviates medially from the normal elbow angle. It usually is secondary to a lateral

Table 5.3 Differential Diagnosis of Elbow Pathology

Disorder	Age (years)	Sex	Swelling	Deformity
Tennis elbow	20–60	Male/Female	No	No
Osteoarthritis	50–80	Female	Yes	Flexion Contractures
Rheumatoid arthritis	5–80+	Female	Yes	Flexion Contractures bilaterally
Cubital tunnel syndrome	20–60	Male/Female	Limited	Possible interosseous and hypothenar wasting

epicondylar fracture and often is present in patients with ulnar nerve palsy.

Note: Better recognition and treatment of supracondylar fractures have made both of these conditions rather infrequent.

The presence of scars can raise the suspicion of motion contractures. Swelling, such as over the olecranon, suggests trauma, infection, foreign body, or bursitis. Limitations in the range of motion (ROM) are sensitive indicators of fracture or other joint pathology:

Flexion	135°
Extension	0°
Supination	90°
Pronation	90°

Palpation

Bony palpation is indicated over the following structures:

- Medial epicondyle,
- Medial supracondylar ridge of humerus,
- Olecranon,
- Ulnar border,
- Olecranon fossa,
- Lateral epicondyle,
- Lateral supracondylar ridge of humerus.

Palpation of soft tissues also is necessary:

- **Medial:** Ulnar nerve and wrist flexor/pronator muscle group, pronator teres, flexor carpi radialis, palmaris longus, flexor carpi ulnaris, medial collateral ligament (MCL), and supracondylar lymph nodes.
- **Posterior:** Olecranon bursa, triceps.
- **Lateral:** Wrist extensors, brachioradialis, extensor carpi radialis longus and brevis, lateral collateral ligaments (LCLs), and annular ligament.
- **Anterior:** Cubical fossa, biceps tendon, brachial artery, median nerve, and musculocutaneous nerve.

Reflexes

Biceps	C5 (C6) via the musculocutaneous nerve
Brachioradialis	C6 (C5) via the radial nerve
Triceps	C7
Absent reflex	Lower motor neuron (LNM) lesion anywhere from C5 root to muscle
Hyperactive reflex	Upper motor neuron (UMN) lesion (the same goes for any hyperreflexive deep tendon reflex)

SPECIAL TESTS

Tested used in the examination of the upper extremity are summarized in Table 5.4.

Elbow Flexion Test

This test is analogous to Phalen's sign in the wrist (**carpal tunnel**) and assesses for numbness and paresthesias caused by ulnar nerve com-

Table 5.4 Common Tests Used in the Examination of the Shoulder

Muscle/Structure	Test
Ulnar nerve/cubital tunnel	Tinel's sign, hypothenar/interosseus wasting
Olecranon bursa, lateral epicondylitis	Tennis elbow test, pain on palpation
Joint laxity	Varus and valgus
Lateral collateral ligament	Pivot shift, varus stress
Medial collateral ligament	Valgus stress, Milkers test

pression in the cubital tunnel. Fully flex both elbows for 30–60 seconds, and ask about sensory changes. A positive test is reproduction of neurologic symptoms with flexion, which indicates ulnar nerve compression.

Ligamentous Stability

This is essentially just a varus and valgus stress test. Apply external and internal stress to the joint of the elbow.

Milker's Test

The Milker's test is shown in Figure 5.3. Instruct the patient to grasp the examiner's thumb and pull downward, as if milking a cow. This maneuver stresses the MCL and reveals MCL weakness. This is a simple and easy test of the MCL, and it should be considered in cases of elbow pain in overhead-throwing athletes.

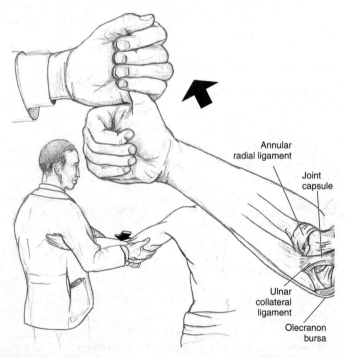

Figure 5.3 Milker's test.

Moving Valgus Stress Test

Place moderate valgus torque on a fully flexed elbow, and then rapidly extend the elbow. A positive test is pain on extension at the medial epicondyle, which indicates MCL laxity or weakness. MCL insufficiency is common in chronically stressed, overhead-throwing athletes.

Pivot Shift Test

This advanced test, as illustrated in Figure 5.4, may be difficult for some practitioners and is not often used. In a supine patient, flex the elbow, supinate the wrist, and apply valgus pressure while also holding the forearm and applying axial pressure. Move through flexion ROM. A positive result is pain, signs of apprehension, or subluxation/dislocation; these imply LCL weakness or tear.

Tennis Elbow Test

In the tennis elbow test (Fig. 5.5), stabilize the forearm while the patient extends it with a fist, and force flexion against the patient's effort. A positive test is pain and paresthesia at the extensor origin of the wrist, which indicates lateral epicondylitis.

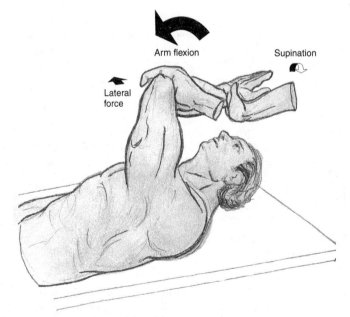

Figure 5.4 Pivot shift test of the elbow.

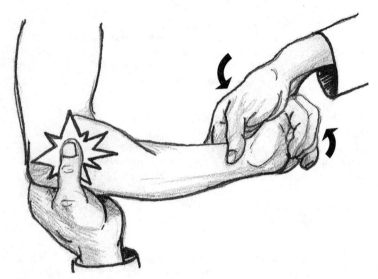

Figure 5.5 Tennis elbow test used to indicate lateral epicondylitis.

Tinel's Sign

Tinel's sign is illustrated in Figure 5.6. Tap or apply pressure at the cubital tunnel; the site is between the medial epicondyle and the olecranon. Tinel's sign is well known in carpal tunnel syndrome, and the symptoms of cubital tunnel syndrome include pain and paresthesias (in this case, in the ulnar nerve distribution).

Valgus Test

Extend the elbow with the wrist supinated. Apply valgus pressure at the elbow and feel for instability, pain, signs of apprehension, or subluxation/dislocation; this indicates MCL instability. Jobe recommended a variation of this test in which the patient places his or her hand in the examiner's axilla while valgus pressure is applied to the elbow.

RADIOLOGIC APPROACH TO THE ELBOW AND FOREARM

Overview

Radiographs of the elbow appear to be either easily visualized or subtle and rather difficult. As always, the clinical examination guides the need for radiography. The ABC'S (**A**lignment, **B**one, **C**artilage, and

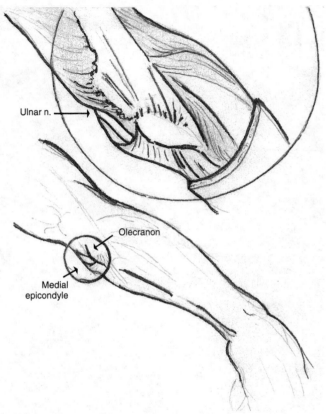

Figure 5.6 Tinel's sign used to indicate cubital tunnel syndrome.

Soft tissue) mnemonic (see Chapter 1) applies to the elbow, where alignment and soft tissue findings may be the only radiographic indicators of injury. Most radiology departments order two standard views: the anteroposterior (AP), and the 90° flexed lateral.

Views

Note: Check to make sure you have the correct patient, the correct date, and the correct anatomy.

Anteroposterior View

The adequate AP radiograph of the elbow shows a fully extended joint without any overlap of bone (Fig. 5.7). Evaluation of bony structures

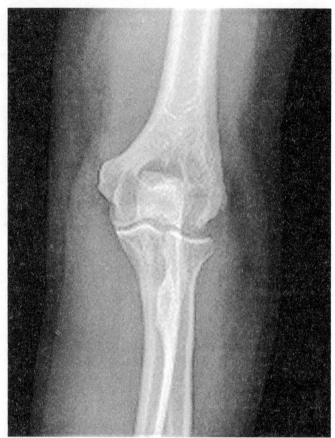

Figure 5.7 Anteroposterior radiograph of the normal elbow.

and cortices for focal disruptions should identify most fractures; however, trabecular impaction may be more difficult to see. Structures to identify are the medial and lateral epicondyles; the lateral condyle (capitellum), which articulates with the radial head; the coronoid process, which articulates with the trochlea; and the supracondylar humerus. Full extension is necessary to prevent radial and capitellar overlap. The radiocapitellar line should be approximated to exclude radial head dislocation, capitellar fractures, and ulnar dislocations. To determine this relationship, a line can be drawn through the radial shaft, which should intersect the capitellum.

Lateral View

For an adequate lateral view (Fig. 5.8), 90° of flexion is necessary. In addition to evaluation of the bony elements, the soft tissue surrounding the anterior and posterior cubital fat pads should always be examined for widening. In many cases, a displaced fat pad is the only evidence of joint effusion and probable intra-articular fracture. Adults are most likely to have a radial head fracture when a fat pad is enlarged, whereas a supracondylar fracture of the humerus is more common in children. The posterior fat pad is a more sensitive indicator of joint pathology, because the anterior fat pad often is present normally. Elbow extension on the lateral radiograph also can produce a view suggesting a false-posterior fat pad.

Structures to identify on the lateral radiograph are the supracondylar humerus, the anterior and posterior fat pads, the olecranon, the radial head, and the coronoid process (Fig. 5.9). The radiocapitel-

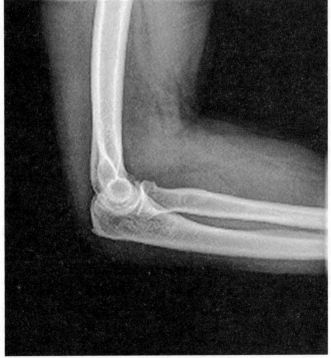

Figure 5.8 Lateral radiograph of the normal elbow.

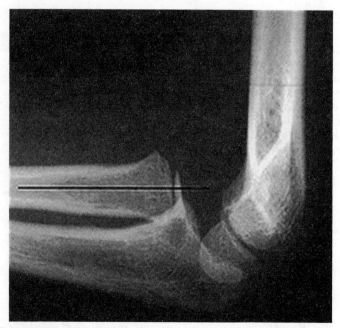

Figure 5.9 Radiograph of anterior humeral line and supracondylar elbow fracture.

lar line should be approximated to exclude radial head dislocation, capitellar fractures, and ulnar dislocations; this relationship should hold for all views. The anterior humeral line can only be estimated on the lateral view and is drawn by continuing the line of the anterior humeral cortex through the middle third of the capitellum (lateral condyle). If this line intersects either the anterior or posterior third of the capitellum, it may indicate a supracondylar elbow fracture.

The Pediatric Elbow

Trauma to the elbow in children is extremely common and often difficult to identify on radiographs because of the presence of secondary centers of ossification if the sequence of ossification is not known to the elevator. Trauma occurs in the following locations according to frequency: supracondylar > lateral condyle > medial epicondyle > radial head. Ossification centers arise and ossify in children beginning shortly after birth and usually ending by puberty (Table 5.5).

Identifying normal centers of ossification can help avoid confusion with fractures. Additionally, before ossification, fracture of carti-

Table 5.5 Ossification of the Immature Elbow

Secondary Ossification Center	Age When It Appears on Radiographs (years)	Approximate Ages Expressed as Odd Numbers
Capitellum	0–1	1
Radial head	3–6	3
Medial epicondyle	3–7	5
Trochlea	7–10	7
Olecranon	8–10	9
Lateral epicondyle	11–12	11

laginous structures is possible and may be evident only by the presence of joint widening, subcapsular hematomas, and disruption of the radiocapitellar and anterior humeral lines. The mechanism of injury and the physical examination are the most important factors in raising the index of suspicion.

SELECTED FRACTURES OF THE ELBOW AND FOREARM

Supracondylar Elbow Fracture

The anatomy of the elbow joint is key to understanding the serious consequences of a supracondylar elbow fracture, which is the most common type of pediatric elbow fracture. The brachial artery follows a posterior course around the olecranon, and the radial, median, and ulnar nerves are all in jeopardy with this injury. The force of a fall on an outstretched arm translates force to the distal humeral head, resulting in a potential lacerating bone fragment. The median nerve is most often injured, followed by the radial nerve and then the ulnar nerve. The brachial artery is associated with a posterolaterally displaced fragment and demands rapid assessment and identification. Compartment syndrome, marked by the five Ps (**P**ain, **P**allor, **P**oikilothermia [cold], **P**aresthesia, and ultimately, **P**ulselessness), can occur when vascular injury leads to increased intracompartmental pressures. Pain with passive extension is the most sensitive indicator of a compartment syndrome and should always be checked.

Initial management should include splinting the injured extremity in a 20° to 30° flexed position. Occult fractures can be easily identified on radiographs, but radiographs also should be scrutinized for other signs of injury, such as the fat pad or "sail sign" (i.e., as a subcapsular hematoma lifts the anterior or posterior fat pad off of the humeral surface). These fractures are graded I–III based on the degree of fragment displacement (I = nondisplaced; II = angulated, with cortex intact; III = displaced). The higher the grade, the more likely are neurovascular complications and injury.

Radial Head Dislocation

Although the name **nursemaids' elbow** may indicate some unfortunate pathology in the arm of a nanny, this name for an elbow dislocation/subluxation actually derives from the injury acquired by the child in the nanny's care. A sharp, forceful pull on an outstretched arm pulls the radial head out of its home in the annular ligament, leaving the child complaining of elbow pain (or pain anywhere between the elbow and hand). The annular ligament then becomes pinched in the elbow joint, often with a tear at its attachment to the radial head. This often leaves the child preferring a position of extension or slight flexion and pronation. This injury is relatively common, occurring mostly between one and three years of age and only rarely after five years. On a lateral flexion radiograph, a line can be drawn through the middle of the radius that should intersect with the capitellum of the humerus.

Treatment focuses on reduction of the subluxed radial head. In a comparative reduction study, wrist hyperpronation was compared with supination at the wrist and elbow flexion; the hyperpronation method was shown to have greater success (95% success rate after the first attempt, and 97.5% with an additional attempt). The traditional method involves applying pressure with the thumb at the radial head, which is then followed by supination at the wrist and elbow flexion to 90°. Either method appears to have good success with reducing the elbow. (See Fig. 4.9, page 94.)

Galeazzi Fracture

A Galeazzi fracture (Fig. 5.10a) is a common fracture pattern that involves a distal radial shaft fracture associated with a distal radioulnar dislocation. A fall on an outstretched arm is the most common mechanism, followed by direct trauma. The most common direction of dislocation is dorsal because of decreased muscle mass in this direction. Nondisplaced fractures are uncommon, and the prospect of a closed reduction is limited and prone to failure. It is important to determine the direction of displacement of the proximal radial fragment on the AP radiograph, because this guides the approach and fixation by the surgeon. More often, the proximal radial fragment is pronated, and the radial tuberosity is directed medially. Otherwise, the radial tuberosity faces laterally, and the proximal fragment is pronated. Open reduction

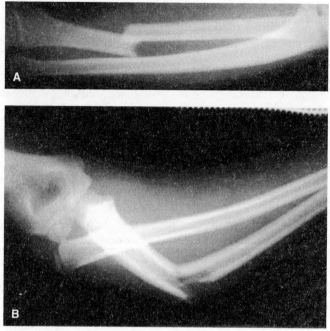

Figure 5.10 Two distinct fractures. **a:** Galeazzi fracture. **b:** Monteggia fracture.

and internal fixation with plates and screws are the preferred treatments. Frequently, the distal radioulnar joint and triangular fibrocartilage ligament complex is repaired or stabilized with Kirschner wires (also known as K-wires) to prevent dorsal instability.

Monteggia's Fracture

The Monteggia's fracture (Fig. 5.10b) involves a fracture of the proximal ulna with a proximal radial head dislocation. There are four grades of this fracture:

- **Type I:** Anterior dislocation of the radial head with a fracture of the ulnar diaphysis.
- **Type II:** Posterior or posterolateral dislocation of the radial head and a posteriorly angulated fracture of the ulnar diaphysis ("reverse Monteggia's fracture").
- **Type III:** Lateral/anterolateral dislocation of the radial head and fracture of the ulnar metaphysis.

- **Type IV:** Fracture of both the radius and ulna, with dislocation of the radial head.

The most common pattern is type I, in which the fracture of the ulna is accompanied by anterior dislocation of the radial head when the elbow joint is in extension. When the elbow is in flexion and the ulna is fractured, posterior dislocation of the radial head is more common.

Medial Epicondyle Flexor Tendon Avulsion Fracture

This type of avulsion fracture deserves mention, because it is one of the few fractures of the elbow that responds well to closed reduction. The AP radiographs of the elbow should be scrutinized for fracture fragments at the medial epicondyle. A trial of conservative, closed reduction therapy should be attempted, and if pain and disability persist, then fixation of the fracture fragment with K-wires can be considered.

Olecranon Fractures

These are very common fractures with a bimodal distribution in the young and old. They can occur either from direct trauma, which can result in significant comminution, or from indirect trauma caused by avulsion of the triceps tendon.

SELECTED DISORDERS OF THE ELBOW AND FOREARM

Lateral Epicondylitis

Often referred to as **tennis elbow,** this repetitive-use injury involves inflammation of the lateral epicondyle at the site of superficial extensor muscles origin. Lateral epicondylitis should be distinguished from medial epicondylitis (**golfer's elbow**), which affects the forearm flexors. It is common in tennis players because of their repetitive, forceful contraction of the common extensor tendon, especially with backhand strokes. Although approximately 10–50% of people who play tennis regularly develop this condition, epicondylitis is not restricted to tennis. This pathology is commonly seen by orthopaedists, and predominantly in people who do not play tennis. Initially an inflammatory condition, the presence of mostly microtears and fibroblastic repair has given lateral epicondylitis the more scientific name of angiofibroblastic tendinosis, a degenerative process. The history and physical examination (see *Basic Exami-*

nation) are key to establishing the diagnosis. Radiography shows calcific pathology in less than 10% of cases, and magnetic resonance imaging often is not helpful. Nonoperative treatment is the preferred approach and is effective in up to 90% of cases. Elimination of the offending movements and use of nonsteroidal anti-inflammatory drugs, with stretching and massage, constitute conservative treatment. Surgical treatment has shown excellent results but is reserved for those who have failed extensive conservative treatment.

Cubital Tunnel Syndrome

Cubital tunnel syndrome occurs when the ulnar nerve is impinged as it passes over the olecranon in the medial epicondylar ulnar groove (cubital tunnel). The ulnar collateral ligament is an essential stabilizer and protector of the ulnar nerve in preventing excessive valgus forces. The impingement results in aching and pain at the medial elbow (the usual presenting symptom). This pathology is common in throwing athletes and is almost always a repetitive stress/overuse injury. Recovery is related to the duration of impingement, and successful treatment is correlated to this factor. Paresthesia in the distribution of the ulnar nerve, extending to the little and ring fingers, often is the presenting symptom, whereas hypothenar and interosseus muscle wasting is a late sign of chronic impingement.

Electromyographic studies can be confirmatory following a good history and physical examination involving elbow flexion. The presence of paresthesias on the dorsum of the hand (ulnar distribution) rules out pathology at the wrist, because sensory nerves penetrate the dorsal hand proximal to the wrist. As with most inflammatory repetitive-use injuries, treatment first focuses on rest and anti-inflammatory medications. When rest fails, there are three principal surgical procedures: decompression, subcutaneous transposition, and submuscular transposition can be performed, depending on the activity and needs of the patient.

Triceps Tendonitis

This disorder commonly occurs, especially in weight lifters who repetitively stress the distal insertion of the triceps tendon at the olecranon. Avulsion fractures also are not uncommon in this group. Painful extension against resistance is evident on examination, and radiographs usually are normal unless chronic calcific tendonitis is present.

Quick Look • Elbow and Forearm

Inspect the skin, looking for such features as gross deformity, guarding, and bruising.

Palpate the soft tissues surrounding the elbow and forearm, especially the olecranon bursa.

Move the elbow through ROM.

- **Elbow flexion:** 135°.
- **Extension:** 0°.
- **Supination:** 90°.
- **Pronation:** 90°.

Reflex testing if neurologic deficits, cervical stenosis, or UMN/LMN disorder is suspected or if the patient is preoperative or postoperative.

- **Biceps (C5), brachioradialis (C6), triceps (C7).**
  - **Absent:** Neuropathy, LMN lesion.
  - **Hyperactive:** UMN lesion.

Evaluate muscles using **special tests** to isolate the disorder.

- **Elbow flexion:** Fully flex both elbows for 30–60°. Do sensory changes occur?
- **Ligamentous stability:** Varus and valgus stress applied to joint of the elbow.
- **Milker's:** Patient grasps the examiner's thumb and pulls downward.
- **Moving valgus stress:** Apply valgus torque on a fully flexed elbow, then rapidly extend the elbow; the patient should not have pain on extension.
- **Pivot shift:** Indicates LCL instability; flex the elbow, supinate the wrist, and apply valgus pressure while also holding the forearm and applying axial pressure. Move through flexion ROM.
- **Tennis elbow:** Force flexion against the patient's effort.
- **Tinel's sign:** Tap or apply pressure at the cubital tunnel.
- **Valgus:** Indicates MCL instability; apply valgus pressure at the elbow, and feel for instability. Does pain occur?

Order appropriate films.

- **AP:** Evaluate bony structures and cortices. Identify the medial and lateral epicondyles, lateral condyle, coronoid process, trochlea, and supracondylar humerus. Approximate the radiocapitellar line.

> • **Lateral:** Evaluate the bony elements. Examine the anterior
> and posterior cubital fat pads for widening. Identify the
> supracondylar humerus, anterior and posterior fat pads,
> olecranon, radial head, and coronoid process. Approxi-
> mate the radiocapitellar line. Estimate the anterior humeral
> line and radiocapitellar line.

SELECTED REFERENCES

Garden RS. Tennis elbow. J Bone Joint Surg Br 1961;43:100–106.

Keefe DT, Lintner DM. Nerve injuries in the throwing elbow. Clin Sports Med 2004;23:723–742.

Macias CG, Bothner J, Wiebe R. A comparison of supination/flexion to hyperpronation in the reduction of radial head subluxations. Pediatrics 1998;102:e10.

Marx JA. Rosen's Emergency Medicine: Concepts and Clinical Practice. 6th Ed. St. Louis: Mosby, 2006.

McDonald J, Whitelaw C, Goldsmith LJ. Radial head subluxation: comparing two methods of reduction. Acad Emerg Med 1999;6:715–718.

Mikic ZD. Galeazzi fracture–dislocations. J Bone Joint Surg Am 1975; 57:1071–1078.

Moore KL. Clinically Oriented Anatomy. 3rd Ed. Baltimore: Williams & Wilkins, 1992.

Morrey BF. Acute and chronic instability of the elbow. J Am Acad Orthop Surg 1996;4:117–128.

O'Driscoll SW, Lawton RL, Smith AM. The "moving valgus stress test" for medial collateral ligament tears of the elbow. Am J Sports Med 2005;33:231–239.

Overly F, Steele DW. Common pediatric fractures and dislocations. Clin Pediatr Emerg Med 2002;3:106–117.

Whaley AL, Baker CL. Lateral epicondylitis. Clin Sports Med 2004; 23:677–691.

6

Wrist and Hand

The bones of the wrist and the hand are shown in Figure 6.1.

ANATOMY

Ulna

The ulna was discussed in detail in Chapter 5.

Radius

The radius was discussed in detail in Chapter 5. An additional term, however, is the **radial styloid,** which is the site of the brachioradialis tendon between the extensor pollicis longus and brevis and is palpable within the anatomic "snuff box." The importance of the snuff box relates to the scaphoid carpal bone, which underlies this space. Fracture of the scaphoid has a high incidence of avascular necrosis and manifests as snuff box tenderness.

Carpals

Anatomically, the bones of the wrist should be memorized. The carpal bones are organized into proximal and distal rows. The proximal row is more important to the function of the wrist, and the radiocarpal is key to wrist movement.

The ligamentous arrangement is complex and, for the average reader, is not high yield. Some exceptions include the space of Poirier and the triangular fibrocartilage complex. The space of Poirier is the interval between the lunate and capitate on the volar aspect of the wrist. This space is lacking significant ligamentous support and has increased susceptibility to carpal dislocations. The triangular fibrocartilage complex consists of several ligaments, including a meniscal homologue and the extensor carpi radialis tendon, which serve to add strength to the distal radioulnar joint (DRUJ).

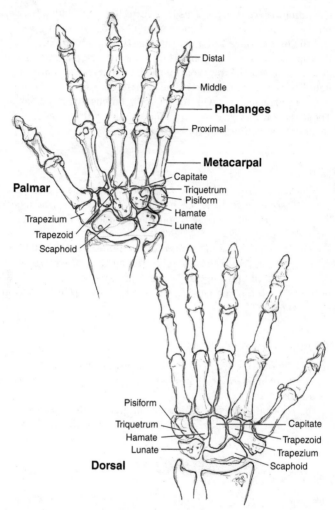

Figure 6.1 Bony upper extremity. All metacarpal and phalangeal bones are organized as head, shaft, and base.

Other joints involving the carpals are:

- **Midcarpal joint:** This is an articulation between the capitate and hamate with the scaphoid lunate and triquetrum. The pisiform bone has no articulation except where it overlies the triquetrum.

- **Carpometacarpal joint:** This joint forms the articulation between the distal carpal row (hamate, capitate, trapezoid, and trapezium) and the first through fifth metacarpals. The thumb articulates with the trapezium as a saddle joint. The second metacarpal has a primary articulation with the trapezoid and also with the trapezium and capitate. The third metacarpal is in line with the capitate only. The fourth metacarpal articulates with the capitate, but also with the hamate. The hamate forms a saddle-type joint with the fifth metacarpal. The second through fourth metacarpals are plane-type synovial joints.

Metacarpals

The metacarpals are homologous with other long bones of greater size and also share their features, each having a base, a shaft, and a head. The heads are oriented distally, opposite the radius. The bases form the knuckles of the fist.

The condyloid joints of the **metacarpophalangeal (MCP) joint** permit motion in two planes. The convex heads of the metacarpals articulate with the phalangeal bases. The larger metacarpal heads accommodate the phalangeal bases better in the frontal (flexion–extension) plane.

Phalanges

Phalanges two through five have three digits, and the thumb has two digits. Cleland and Grayson's ligaments secure the skin to the fingers for manual dexterity.

The **interphalangeal joints** are uniplanar hinge joints. They are supported by lateral collateral ligaments and a palmar ligament (Figure 6.2).

Muscles

Table 6.1 presents information about the muscles of the forearm and their nerves/roots, and Table 6.2 outlines the basic muscular organization of the wrist and hand. Evaluate using the pinch test (discussed later). Long flexors and extensors stabilize the interphalangeal joints, the MCP joints, and the carpometacarpal joints and create arch. The interossei create pinch.

Vascular Anatomy

Figure 6.3 shows the location of the major arteries and nerves of the hand.

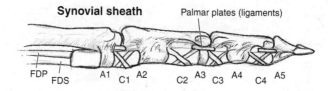

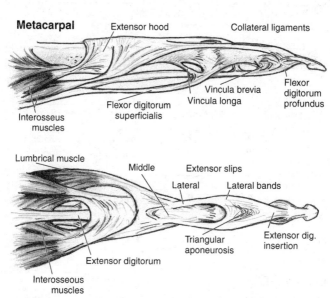

Figure 6.2 The volar surface of the distal radioulnar joint (DRUJ). A, annular; C, cruciform; dig., digitorum; FDP, flexor digitorum profundus; FDS, flexor digitorum superficialis.

Wrist Fascial Zones

The wrist tunnels are separate fascial structures (Fig. 6.4), which are of clinical importance in traumatic tendon repairs. The tunnel of Guyon travels through the hook of the hamate and transmits the ulnar nerve and artery.

The other wrist tunnels are:

- **Tunnel 1:** Site of stenosing tenosynovitis (DeQuervain's disease).
- **Tunnel 2:** Extensor carpus radialis longus and extensor carpus radialis brevis are at the radial side of the tubercle.

Table 6.1 Muscles of the Forearm and Their Nerves/Roots

Muscle	Nerve (Root)	Origin	Insertion
Lower arm			
Pronator teres	Median nerve (C6 and C7)	Medial epicondyle and coronoid process	Volar and proximal radius
Flexor carpi radialis	Median nerve (C6 and C7)	Medial epicondyle	Second metacarpal base
Palmaris longus	Median nerve (C7 and C8)	Medial epicondyle	Flexor retinaculum and palmar aponeurosis
Flexor carpi ulnaris	Median nerve (C7 and C8)	Medial epicondyle Olecranon and dorsal ulna	Hook of hamate, pisiform, and fifth metacarpal
Flexor digitorum superficialis	Median nerve (C7, C8, and T1)	Medial epicondyle, coronoid process, and ulnar collateral ligament Volar radius	Phalanges 2–5
Deep forearm flexors			
Flexor digitorum profundus	Medial aspect ulnar nerve Lateral aspect median v	Medial and anterior ulna	Base of phalanges 2–5
Flexor pollicis longus	Anterior interosseus nerve (C8 and T1)	Anterior radius and interosseus membrane	Base of thumb
Pronator quadratus	Anterior interosseus nerve (C8 and T1)	Distal anterior ulna	Distal anterior radius

Table 6.1 Muscles of the Forearm and Their Nerves/Roots *(Continued)*

Muscle	Nerve (Root)	Origin	Insertion
Forearm extensors			
Brachioradialis	Radial nerve (C5, C6, and C7)	Lateral supra-condylar humerus	Lateral and distal radius
Extensor carpi radialis longus	Radial nerve (C6 and C7)	Lateral supra-condylar humerus	Base of fifth metacarpal
Extensor carpi radialis brevis	Deep radial nerve (C7 and C8)	Lateral epicondyle	Base of third metacarpal
Extensor digitorum	Posterior interosseus nerve (C7 and C8)	Lateral epicondyle	Extensor expansion at digits 2–5
Extensor digiti minimi	Posterior interosseus nerve (C7 and C8)	Lateral epicondyle	Extensor expansion at fifth digit
Extensor carpi ulnaris	Posterior interosseus nerve (C7 and C8)	Lateral epi-condyle and posterior ulna	Base of fifth metacarpal

Table 6.2 Muscles of the Wrist and Hand

Muscle	Nerve (Root)	Origin	Insertion
Wrist extension	C6		
Extensor carpi radialis longus	Radial nerve (C6 and C7)	Lateral supra-condylar ridge	Base of third metacarpal
Extensor carpi radialis brevis	Radial nerve (C6 and C7)	Lateral epicondyle	Base of third metacarpal
Extensor carpi ulnaris	Radial nerve (C6 and C7)	Lateral epicondyle	Base of fifth metacarpal

(continued on next page)

Table 6.2 Muscles of the Wrist and Hand *(Continued)*

Muscle	Nerve (Root)	Origin	Insertion
Wrist flexion	C7		
Flexor carpi radialis	Median nerve (C7)	Medial epi-condyle	Base of second and third metacarpals
Flexor carpi ulnaris	Ulnar nerve (C8 and T1)	Medial epicondyle, olecranon, and ulna	Hook of hamate and base of fifth metacarpal
Finger extension			
Extensor digito-rum communis	Radial nerve (C7)	Lateral epicondyle	Extensor expansion 2–5 digits
Extensor indicis	Radial nerve (C7)	Posterior ulna	Second digit of distal phalanx
Extensor digiti minimi	Radial nerve (C7)	Lateral epicondyle	Fifth digit of distal phalanx
Finger flexion	C8		
Distal inter-phalangeal			
Flexor digitorum profundus	Ulnar nerve (C8 and T1)	Proximal, medial, and anterior ulna	Base of distal pha-langes 2–5
Proximal inter-phalangeal			
Flexor digitorum superficialis	Median nerve (C7, C8, and T1)	Medial epicondyle and superior anterior radius	Middle phalanx digits 2–5
Flexor digiti minimi brevis	Deep ulnar (C8 and T1)	Hook of hamate and flexor retinaculum	Medial fifth bone

Table 6.2 Muscles of the Wrist and Hand *(Continued)*

Muscle	Nerve (Root)	Origin	Insertion
Metacarpo-phalangeal (flexors)			
Lumbricals		Lateral aspect of flexor digitorum profundus tendons	Lateral extensor expansion
Medial two	Ulnar nerve (C8)		
Lateral two	Median nerve (C7)		
Finger abduction	T1		
Dorsal interossei	Ulnar nerve (C8 and T1)	Dorsal sides of metacarpals	Extensor expansion digits 2–4
Abductor digiti minimi	Ulnar nerve (C8 and T1)	Base of pisiform	Medial base of fifth digit
Finger adduction	T1		
Palmar interossei	Ulnar nerve (C8 and T1)	Medial palmar base of digits 2, 4, and 5	Extensor expansion digits 2, 4, and 5
Thumb extension			
Metacarpo-phalangeal			
Extensor pollicis brevis	Radial nerve (C7)	Posterior radius	Base of proximal thumb
Extensor pollicis longus	Radial nerve (C7)	Posterior ulna and radius	Base of distal thumb
Thumb flexion			
Metacarpo-phalangeal			
Flexor pollicis brevis		Flexor retinaculum, trapezium	Base of proximal thumb
Medial aspect	Ulnar nerve (C8)		
Lateral aspect	Median nerve (C6 and C7)		

(continued on next page)

Muscle	Nerve (Root)	Origin	Insertion
Flexor pollicis longus	Median nerve (C8 and T1)	Anterior radius and interosseus membrane	Base of thumb
Thumb abduction			
Abductor pollicis longus	Radial nerve (C7)	Posterior radius and ulna	Lateral base of proximal thumb
Abductor pollicis brevis	Median nerve (C6 and C7)	Flexor retinaculum, scaphoid, and trapezium	
Thumb adduction			
Adductor pollicis	Ulnar nerve (C8)	Oblique head: Bases of the second and third metacarpals, capitate, Transverse head: Palmar third metacarpal	Medial base of proximal thumb
Opposition			
Opponens pollicis	Median nerve (C6 and C7)	Flexor retinaculum and trapezium	Lateral first metacarpal
Opponens digiti minimi	Ulnar nerve (C8)	Hook of hamate and flexor retinaculum	Medial fifth metacarpal

Table 6.2 Muscles of the Wrist and Hand *(Continued)*

- **Tunnel 3:** Extensor pollicis longus, ulnar border of snuff box, makes a 45° turn over the extensor carpus radialis longus and extensor carpus radialis brevis.
- **Tunnel 4.** Extensor digitorum communis and extensor indicis.
  - Common site of ganglion cysts.
  - Ulnar styloid; look for ulnar styloid process fracture often with a Colles' fracture.

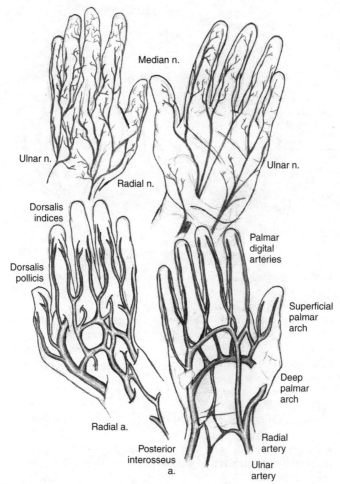

Figure 6.3 Vascular anatomy of the hand. a., artery; n., nerve.

- **Tunnel 5:** Extensor digiti minimi.
- **Tunnel 6:** Extensor carpi ulnaris.

Hand Zones

The hand is divided into several zones:

- **Thenar eminence:** The full muscular pad of the palm connected to the base of the thumb. This prominence can atrophy with chronic carpal tunnel syndrome. It involves three muscles:

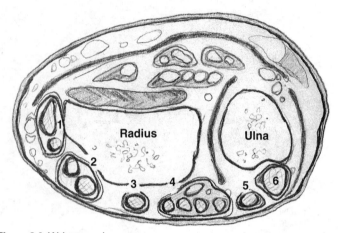

Figure 6.4 Wrist tunnels.

- Abductor pollicis brevis.
- Opponens pollicis.
- Flexor pollicis brevis.
- **Hypothenar eminence:** This lesser prominence of the palm is part of the base of the fifth digit. The hypothenar eminence can atrophy with chronic ulnar nerve compression (cubital tunnel syndrome). It also involves three muscles:
  - Abductor digiti quinti.
  - Opponens digiti.
  - Flexor digiti quinti.
- **Palm:** Items of the palm that are pertinent to the examination include:
  - Palmer fascia/aponeurosis.
  - Finger flexor tendons travel in a common sheath.
- **Dorsum of the hand:** Contains no muscle bellies, only tendons. In rheumatoid arthritis, extensor tendons are ulnar displaced/deviated at the MCP joint.
- **Phalanges:** In osteoarthritis, there is nodular enlargement at proximal interphalangeal (PIP) and distal interphalangeal (DIP) joints.

Figures 6.5, 6.6, and 6.7 show the boutonnière, mallet finger, and swan-neck deformities, respectively. Table 6.3 provides more information about these conditions.

BASIC EXAMINATION

A complete assessment of the hand is, unfortunately, beyond the scope of this book. Instead, the basic examination should focus on the "great-

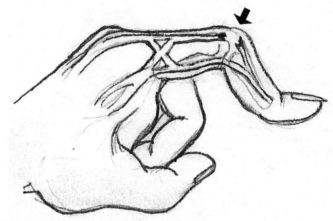

Figure 6.5 Boutonnière deformity.

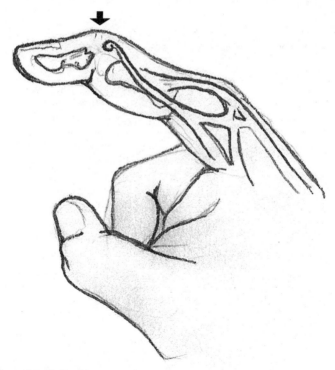

Figure 6.6 Mallet finger.

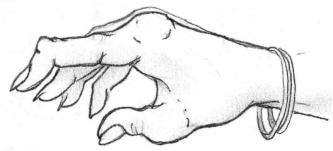

Figure 6.7 Swan-neck deformity.

est hits" of hand tests, such as the Phalen's and Tinel's signs for carpal tunnel syndrome and Kanavel signs for infection below (Table 6.4):

1. Fingers held in flexion.
2. Uniform swelling.

Table 6.3 Selected Deformities of the Wrist and Hand

Condition	Description
Swan neck	Proximal interphalangeal (PIP) hyperextension; distal interphalangeal (DIP) flexion
Z	Hyperextension of the interphalangeal joint; fixed flexion and subluxation of the metacarpophalangeal (MCP) joint
Boutonniere	Avulsion of extensor digitorum communis at insertion of middle phalanx; increased PIP flexion
Volkmann's	Flexion contracture involving one to all digits of the hand secondary to ischemia (compartment syndrome)
Mallet	Avulsion fracture of extensor digitorum communis; ends of fingers
Ruptured extensor slip	Boutonniere or mallet
Paronychia	"Hangnail" infection of lateral border of nail bed
Felon	Deep infection of finger pads
Heberden's nodes	DIP enlargement indicative of osteoarthritis
Bouchard's nodes	Fusiform enlargement at MCP and PIP

Table 6.4 Common Tests Used in Examination of the Wrist and Hand

Muscle/Structure	Test
Median nerve/carpal tunnel	Tinel's sign and Phalen's sign, digital compression test
Joint contracture versus muscle tightness	Bunnel-Littler test
Retinacular contracture versus joint capsule tightness	Retinacular test
Tenosynovitis	Kanavel signs and Finkelstein test
Lunotriquetral ligament	Regan test
Scapholunate interosseus ligament	Watson test

3. Pain on passive extension.
4. Pain on palpation of tendon sheaths.

Note: So-called snuff box tenderness should not be missed, and the risk factors for degenerative and rheumatoid joint disease should be considered in the differential diagnosis (Table 6.5).

Visual Examination

Palmer Surface

The palmar surface of the hand should first be examined for gross deformity, loss of symmetry, and swelling of focal nodules or lesions.

Table 6.5 Differential Diagnosis of Hand Pathology

Disorder	Age (years)	Sex	Deformity
Carpal tunnel syndrome	40–80	Males and females	Thenar atrophy
Osteoarthritis	50–80	Females	Flexion and lateral deviation of proximal interphalangeal and distal interphalangeal; Heberden's nodes
Rheumatoid arthritis	50–80+	Females	Flexion of metacarpophalangeal and proximal interphalangeal, ulnar deviation (swan neck), and boutonnière

The general shape of the fingers should be appreciated; for instance, short stubby fingers are seen in achondroplasia, acromegaly, and hyperparathyroidism. The fusiform swelling of "sausage digits" accompanies the presentation of psoriatic arthritis. Hypertrophy of individual digits occurs in neurofibromatosis and Paget's disease as well as in trauma (collateral ligament tears) and rheumatoid arthritis. The general location of arthritic involvement can be a rough guide for differentiating rheumatoid arthritis from osteoarthritis. Rheumatoid arthritis can first be picked up as unusual moist and sticky hands, which later develop painful swelling and deformation at the MCP and PIP joints.

Dorsal Surface

Repeat the assessment as described for the palmar surface above. Figures 6.8 and 6.9 illustrate felon and paronychia, respectively.

Palpation

The radial styloid process, anatomic snuff box, navicular, trapezium, radial tubercle (Lister's tubercle), capitate, lunate, ulnar styloid process,

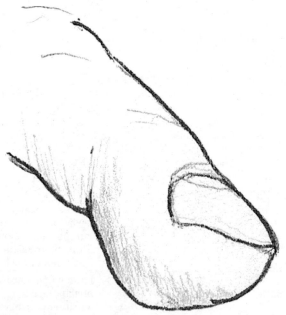

Figure 6.8 Felon.

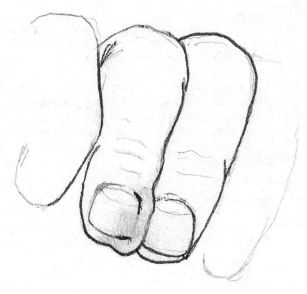

Figure 6.9 Paronychia.

triquetrum, pisiform, hook of hamate, metacarpals, first metacarpal, MCP joint, and phalanges should be palpated. The wrist and hand should be taken through a standard examination exhibiting range of motion (ROM) to major areas of the hand:

Wrist flexion	90°
Wrist extension	75–90°
Radial deviation	10–30°
Ulnar deviation	10–30°
MCP	0–90°
PIP	0–100°
DIP	0–80°
Thumb interphalangeal flexion	80°
Thumb interphalangeal extension	20°

The sequence of moving the hand and digits through the ROM is individual. A more detailed hand examination can be performed if necessary or if your specialty demands it. A simple neurologic examination of the hand also should be done, noting the cutaneous sensation that corresponds to the distal innervation of the upper extremity (see Figure 6.22). Isolation of the individual nerves is outlined in *Special Tests.*

SPECIAL TESTS

Allen Test

The Allen test provides an indication of radial artery versus ulnar artery sufficiency. Ask the patient to squeeze his or her hand several times to milk blood out of the hand and then hold a fist while the examiner occludes the radial, and then the ulnar, artery. In both instances, the hand should quickly flush and reperfuse when the patient opens the fist. This test works well for assessing digital artery perfusion.

Bunnel-Littler Test

The Bunnel-Littler test (Fig. 6.10) distinguishes between phalangeal intrinsic muscle tightness and joint capsule contracture. If, with some attempt to flex the PIP joint, there is no flexion, the patient has tight intrinsics or joint capsule contracture. Next, instruct the patient to flex at the MCP joint. If patient can flex now, he or she has tight intrinsics; if there is no flexion, the patient has capsule contracture.

Carpal Tunnel Compression Test

Apply direct pressure with your thumb to the palm, close to the wrist between the thenar and hypothenar eminences. Reproduction of paresthesias is sensitive for carpal tunnel syndrome.

Elson's Test

The Elson's test (Fig. 6.11) indicates a ruptured central tendon slip. The extensor mechanism of the finger can be injured when "jammed"

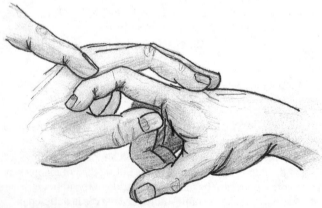

Figure 6.10 Bunnel-Littler test.

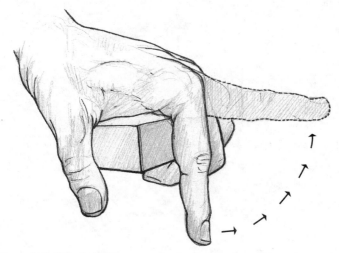

Figure 6.11 Elson's test.

or in sudden flexion injuries. Have the patient rest his or her finger at the PIP joint at the edge of the examination table. Instruct the patient to extend the finger while it is immobilized on the table. A positive test is extension at the PIP joint; if such extension is compromised, then the middle slip is ruptured. If the middle slip is intact but the lateral bands are ruptured, then the DIP joint is nonfunctional, and this results in a boutonnière deformity.

Finkelstein Test

The Finkelstein test (Fig. 6.12) indicates tenosynovitis. The patient makes a fist with the thumb tucked in and ulnar flexes the wrist. A positive test is pain reduction in tunnel 1, indicating DeQuervain's disease (tenosynovitis).

Froment Test

The Froment test indicates ulnar nerve neuropathy. Instruct the patient to pinch a piece of paper. A weak pinch at the DIP joint of the thumb implies ulnar neuropathy.

Opposition Test

The opposition test indicates median neuropathy. The patient pinches using the thumb and little finger. A positive test is weakness involving the opponens pollicis.

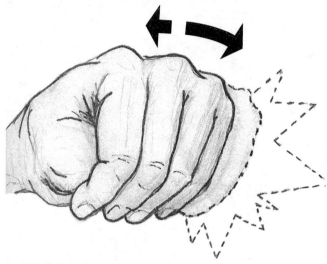

Figure 6.12 Finkelstein test.

Phalen's Sign

The Phalen's sign (Fig. 6.13) indicates carpal tunnel syndrome. Use bilateral volar wrist flexion for 30 to 60 seconds to elicit pain and/or paresthesia in sensory distribution.

Pinch Test

The pinch test indicates weakness of the flexor pollicis longus. The patient pinches with the thumb and index finger. A positive test is the inability to maintain pinch grip (anterior interosseous neuropathy, deep branch of the median nerve).

Regan Test

The Regan test indicates a lunotriquetral ligament tear. Stabilize the lunate while manipulating the ulnar aspect of the wrist, feeling for instability.

Retinacular Test

The retinacular test distinguishes between retinacular tightness and capsule contracture. Flex the DIP while holding the PIP. A positive test is no flexion at the DIP. Then, flex the finger at the PIP and try again. If flexion now occurs, then the patient has retinacular tightness. If flexion still does not occur, then the patient has contracture.

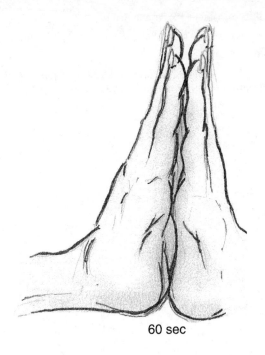

60 sec

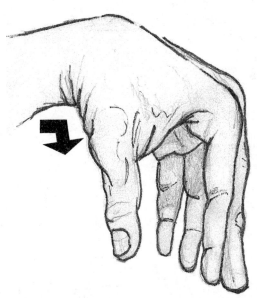

Figure 6.13 Phalen's sign.

Tinel's Sign

The Tinel's sign (Fig. 6.14) indicates carpal tunnel syndrome. Tap directly over the median (or other peripheral) nerve to elicit pain and/or paresthesia in sensory distribution.

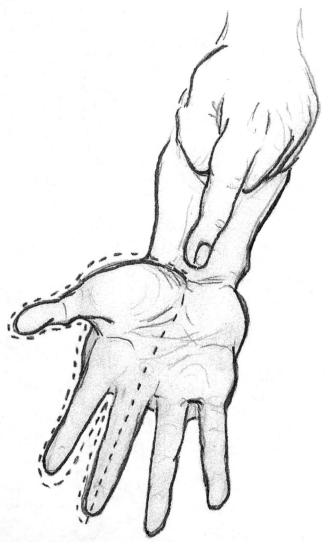

Figure 6.14 Tinel's sign.

Watson Test

The Watson test (Fig. 6.15) indicates a scapholunate interosseus ligament tear. Palpate the volar aspect of the scaphoid. Begin with dorsiflexion and ulnar deviation, then radially deviate the volar wrist flex. If this produces a "clunk" as the lunate moves past the scaphoid, then the patient has some scapholunate pathology.

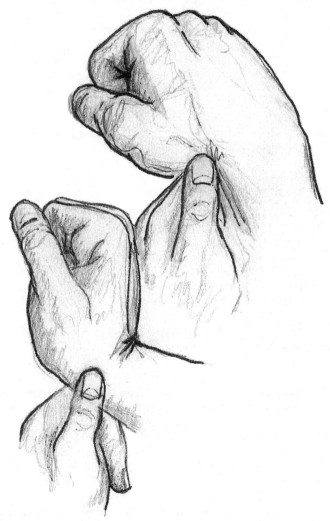

Figure 6.15 Watson test.

RADIOLOGIC APPROACH TO THE WRIST

Overview

Evaluation of wrist radiographs probably is the best example of the benefit that a firm understanding of normal anatomy and radiologic appearance can be to the clinician. The patient history and physical examination often are vague and unrevealing in cases of wrist injuries, but distal radius fractures are easy to detect. The mechanism of injury is always important; however, the majority of wrist injuries occurs after a fall on an outstretched arm. Three standard views are obtained: posteroanterior (PA), lateral, and oblique. The ulnar stressed (scaphoid) view is another common radiograph that should be obtained if a scaphoid fracture is suspected or snuff box tenderness is present.

Views

Note: Check to make sure you have the correct patient, the correct date, and the correct anatomy.

Posteroanterior View

In an adequate PA radiograph, the third metacarpal should line up with the radial shaft. The lunate overlies the DRUJ, and there should be no radial or ulnar deviation. Proper alignment reveals two carpal arcs in the atraumatic wrist, which should be identified in every PA radiograph (Fig. 6.16).

This arrangement is focally disturbed in carpal dislocation. Lunate and perilunate dislocations comprise the great majority. Figure 6.17 displays the carpal bones.

To properly evaluate the distal radius and ulna, 5–6 cm of forearm should be included in the film. Other aspects of evaluating a PA radiograph are:

- The distal radius is commonly fractured and should be scrutinized. The ulnar styloid always should be examined for fracture, especially in cases with a radial fracture.
- Identify the greater and lesser arcs. Look for a gap of more than 4 mm in the scapholunate interval (Terry-Thomas and David Letterman both have a gap in their front teeth), which indicates scapholunate dissociation. All intercarpal distances should be uniform and average 1–2 mm.
- A radiopaque ring on the distal pole of the scaphoid indicates movement (rotary subluxation).

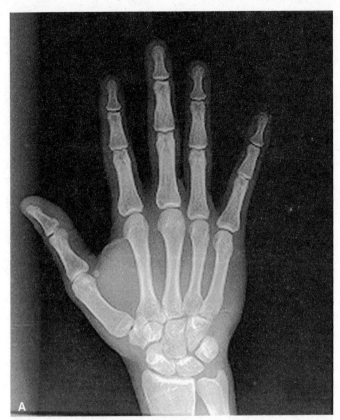

Figure 6.16 a: Radiograph of carpal bones.
(continued on next page)

- Scrutinize the scaphoid bone for fracture, because this is an area of high disability in patients and of high liability to physicians. Use of a hot light can identify a thin (normal) fat stripe along the radial margin of the scaphoid. Increased width of this marker can indicate scaphoid fracture. Obtain ulnar stressed views if fracture is suspected.
- The lunate should be trapezoidal, not triangular. If the lunate is triangular, evaluate for adequacy of the view (i.e., no rotation) or dislocation.

Lateral View

This is a difficult view, showing considerable overlap of the carpal bones; however, this angle offers a clear view of the distal radius and

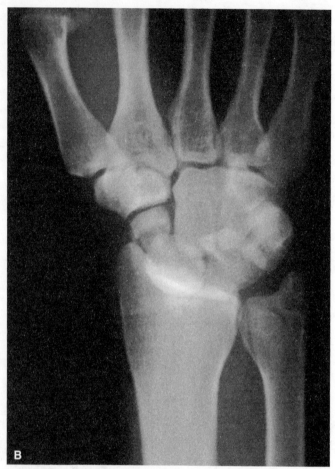

Figure 6.16 *(continued)* **b:** Posteroanterior radiograph of arcs.

ulna. This view is the only one that is used to evaluate for volar or dorsal intercalated segmental instability. For an adequate projection, there should be no flexion or extension at the wrist. The ulnar shaft should overlap the dorsal half of the radius, and the metacarpals and radius should be parallel.

Proper evaluation of a lateral radiograph involves:

• The cortices of the distal radius and ulna should be carefully examined for fracture or focal disruption.

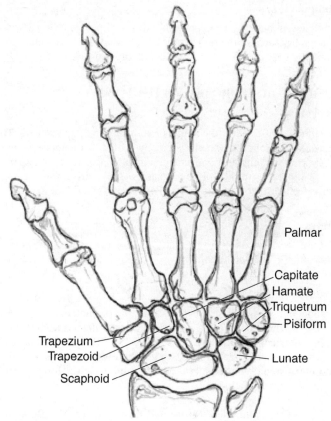

Figure 6.17 Carpal bones.

- Four vertically oriented arcs should be identified. These arcs are created by the articular surface of the radius, the superior and inferior margins of the lunate, and the base of the capitate. The capitate should sit in the cup of the lunate, which should smoothly articulate with the distal radius.
- The scapholunate angle should be assessed. This relationship is created by drawing intersecting lines through the longitudinal axes of the scaphoid and lunate (normal, 30–60°).
- Scan the dorsal cortex of the triquetrum for a chip fracture, which is common.
- The pronator quadratus fat stripe should be seen extending thinly down the volar aspect of the distal radius. Enlargement of the marker can indicate a distal radial fracture.

Oblique View

This view is best for supplementing evaluation of the radial wrist. Oblique fractures of the radius may be apparent. This projection also offers the best view of the trapezoid and trapezium.

RADIOLOGIC APPROACH TO THE HAND

Overview

In contrast to the wrist, the hand is relatively simple to evaluate. The decision to obtain radiographs is largely guided by the mechanism of injury, patient complaint, and examination findings. In addition to fracture, radiographs may be ordered to assess for arthritis, foreign body, or gas from microbial infiltration (as in osteomyelitis).

Views

Note: Check to make sure you have the correct patient, the correct date, and the correct anatomy.

Posteroanterior View

An adequate PA radiograph shows all digits, metacarpals, carpal bones, and the DRUJ. This is a standard view for detecting metacarpal and phalangeal fractures. Always assess the DRUJ and carpal arcs/bones while assessing the digits. **All hand views should assess digit and metacarpal cortices, trabeculae, and articulations.** Specific points of interest include:

- Base of the thumb and fourth and fifth metacarpals (Bennett's, Rolando's, and boxer's fractures).
- Distal radius, DRUJ, and ulnar styloid.
- Scaphoid.
- Metacarpal base, shaft, neck, and heads.

Lateral View

In the lateral radiograph (Fig. 6.18), the distal radius and ulna, as well as the metacarpals, should overlap. The thumb and phalanges, however, should not. This view is good for detecting fractures at the interphalangeal joint.

Oblique View (Pronation)

Some overlap of the metacarpal bases is permissible. The second and third metacarpals should be distinct.

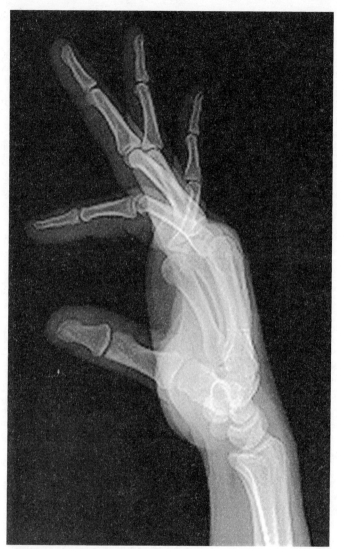

Figure 6.18 Lateral radiograph of the hand.

Oblique View (Supination)

Bilateral comparison of the hands, especially at the fifth digits, make this additional view occasionally worth obtaining in cases of arthritis.

SELECTED FRACTURES OF THE WRIST AND HAND

Colles' Fracture

The Colles' fracture (Fig. 6.19) is the classic upper extremity fracture produced by a fall on an outstretched hand. The resulting dinner-fork deformity is from volar angulation with radial and dorsal displacement of the distal fragment. Often, however, the term is used to describe any distal radial fracture following a fall on the outstretched arm. Treatment is directed at reduction and casting of the break but can include open reduction and internal fixation (ORIF) of the fragment. It is termed an extra-articular fracture of the distal radius, and it does not extend into the joint space. When assessing a distal radius fracture, it is important to inspect the distal ulna as well, because this fracture is frequently associated with fracture of the ulnar styloid.

Smith's Fracture

This is a reverse Colles' fracture, consisting of a dorsally angulated distal radial fragment with a volarly displaced distal fragment.

Scaphoid Fracture

With its key role in articulating with the radius, the scaphoid is especially prone to fracture; it is the most commonly fractured carpal bone. Unfortunately, its vascular supply, via the scaphoid branch of the radial artery, is not always adequate for good healing. Avascular necrosis may occur if good approximation of fracture fragments is not achieved. The body of the scaphoid is kidney-shaped, with a proximal and a distal pole and a thinner midsection, which is termed the *waist*. The waist is the most common site of fracture.

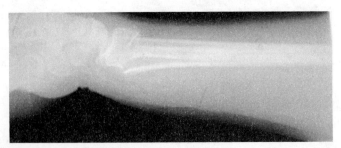

Figure 6.19 Colles' fracture.

Treatment of stable, nondisplaced fractures is immobilization in a thumb spica cast for 6–8 weeks. A displacement of more than 1 mm, a cortical step-off that increases with scapholunate angulation of greater than 60°, or lunatocapitate angulation of more than 15° requires intervention. ORIF can be achieved via Kirschner wires (K-wires) or newer, double-compressive screws that draw the fracture fragments toward each other.

Carpal Dislocations

The typical mechanism of injury for fractures and dislocations of the wrist (Fig. 6.20) is a fall on an outstretched hand. Swelling and localized tenderness are sensitive indicators of injury. The radial margin (scaphoid and trapezium) and proximal row (scaphoid, lunate, and triquetrum) are the most susceptible to injury. The radius, lunate, and capitate are all in the sagittal plane and have been conceptualized as a central link of stability. Disruption of the scaphoid in this arrangement often pitches the triquetrum, dorsally dislocating it, and the scapholunate angle increases to greater than 70°. If the lunate is fractured or the lunotriquetral ligament complex is disrupted, then the triquetrum is pitched volarly, and volar instability–dislocation ensues.

Gamekeeper's Thumb

Repeated injury to the ulnar collateral ligament can lead to laxity and instability of the thumb MCP joint. These injuries are classified on a scale of 1 to 4 (Table 6.6). They can occur traumatically from a fall on an outstretched, thumb-abducted hand, especially in sports (e.g., ski-pole injury is now most common). Injuries to other structures, such as the volar plates, are likely.

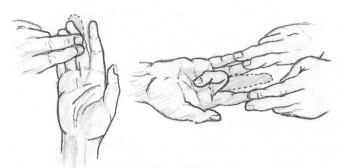

Figure 6.20 Dorsal-volar intercalated segmental instability.

Table 6.6 Classification of Gamekeeper's Thumb

Type	Injury
1	Nondisplaced avulsion fracture of the ulnar collateral ligament
2	Displaced avulsion fracture
3	Torn ligament (stable)
4	Torn ligament (unstable in flexion)

Bennett's/Rolando's Fracture

These two fractures both involve the metacarpal base of the thumb. Fractures of the second through fourth metacarpals often are minimally displaced. Both the Bennett and Rolando patterns are intra-articular fracture–dislocations of the base of the first metacarpal/trapezial joint. They are difficult fractures to reduce and treat. The Bennet pattern is a linear fracture of the volar lip of the thumb base, and the Rolando pattern is comminuted, indicating that forces are greater in the Rolando's fracture.

Treatment is closed reduction with K-wires or ORIF if the displacement is significant. If the palmar and dorsally displaced fragments of a Rolando's fracture are large enough, the surgeon may elect to perform an ORIF with small lag screws incorporated through a shaped buttress plate.

Boxer's Fracture

The boxer's fracture is fracture of the fifth metacarpal neck; as the name implies, this injury is common to fighters, however, not boxers who are trained to hit without angulation. The fifth metacarpal ranks first among metacarpal fractures, followed by base fractures of the thumb (Bennett's and Rolando's). Although swelling makes assessment difficult, neurovascular checks are necessary using cap refill and two-point discrimination before and after manipulation. Fixation with K-wires is necessary if good reduction and approximation are impossible; otherwise, splinting and rest are sufficient.

SELECTED DISORDERS OF THE WRIST AND HAND
Carpal Tunnel Syndrome

This repetitive-use injury may affect people in trades involving heavy use of the wrist and hand (e.g., casino dealer, haircutter or barber, and typist). Entrapment of the median nerve in the carpal tunnel beneath the flexor retinaculum of the wrist results in characteristic symptoms. Thenar atrophy is a late sign. Pain and paresthesias are produced by impingement and are reproduced by the Tinel's and Phalen's signs in the distribution of the median nerve.

Ganglion Cyst

Localized synovial fluid accumulation is the etiology of ganglion cysts. These cysts most often are located in the tendon sheath of the volar and dorsal wrist as well as in the dorsal DIP joint. The location suggests overuse injury as a probable cause, although in some cases, rheumatoid arthritis also has been implicated. Women are affected much more frequently than men.

Treatment is rest with splinting and aspiration if excessively large and restricting of ROM. Recalcitrant cases may require excision, although recurrence is a very common problem.

DeQuervain's Disease

DeQuervain's disease refers to tendonitis of the thumb extensor tendons (abductor pollicis longus and extensor pollicis brevis) and first dorsal compartment swelling. This leads to pain on the volar, thumb side of the wrist, which may be accompanied by a ganglion or a snapping feeling when the tendon catches with thumb movement. DeQuervain's disease is diagnosed via the Finkelstein test, in which the patient makes a fist with the thumb tucked in and the hand tilted toward the middle finger and flexes the wrist. Conservative treatment begins with nonsteroidal anti-inflammatory drugs (NSAIDs) but can involve surgical release of the tendon sheath as well.

Dupuytren's Contracture

This deforming contracture of the hand results from fibrous thickening (fibroblast proliferation and collagen deposition) of the palmar fascia. Possibly hereditary, it has no clear etiology. In some cases, it has occurred in association with cancer, promotion of growth factors, and Northern European ancestry. It is benign but can be disabling, with flexion curling of the fingers. The onset and course are slow, and the ring finger most commonly is affected. The index finger and thumb typically are spared.

Treatment is saved for disabling stages and involves surgery when the MCP joint contracture is 30° or more. Surgical removal of scar tissue is very effective, and recurrence is low.

Trigger Finger (Stenosing Tenosynovitis)

When the tendon sheath that surrounds the phalangeal flexor tendon becomes inflamed, it restricts the action of the finger, most often at the A1 pulley near the PIP joint. The name derives from the catching of the finger in a bent "trigger" position. Trigger finger is a catching or snapping of the flexor digitorum profundus/flexor digitorum superficialis (Fig. 6.21).

Trigger finger is most common in the middle and ring fingers as well as in the thumb. Repetitive stress trauma or general medical conditions, including rheumatoid arthritis, diabetes, hypothyroidism, amyloidosis, and infection, can precipitate the condition. It is very common and is corrected conservatively, with splinting, NSAIDs, or corticosteroid injection. It also can be easily corrected with a surgical release of the A1 tendinous pulley.

Osteoarthritis Versus Rheumatoid Arthritis

Table 6.7 outlines the similarities and differences between these two types of arthritis.

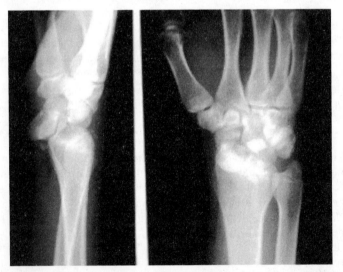

Figure 6.21 Differentiating flexor digitorum superficialis and flexor digitorum profundus.

Table 6.7 Comparison of Osteoarthritis and Rheumatoid Arthritis

Osteoarthritis	Rheumatoid Arthritis
Noninflammatory	Inflammatory
External forces/degenerative	Autoimmune process
Heberden's (distal interphalangeal) and Bouchard's (proximal interphalangeal)	Swan neck/boutonnière; atlantoaxial subluxation
Alkaline phosphatase, +/− elevated	Positive rheumatoid factor (70% IgM anti-IgG), positive C3, positive erythrocyte sedimentation rate, positive antinuclear antibody, and polyclonal gammopathy
Asymmetric involvement, joint space narrowing osteophytes, and eburnation subchondral bone cysts on radiography	Symmetric, joint space narrowing, pannus formation, and ankylosis
Morning pain that decreases with activity	No circadian variation
Diagnosis via history, physical, and radiologic findings	Diagnosis via history, physical, and laboratory findings
Treatment with nonsteroidal anti-inflammatory drugs	Treatment with methotrexate; physical therapy to prevent ankylosis

Kienböck's Disease

Proximal carpal row collapse is thought to result from wrist trauma (usually forgotten loading or repetitive fractures), which then leads to vascular insufficiency of the lunate bone. Eventual avascular necrosis and collapse of the bone results in wrist pain radiating up the forearm and stiffness or weakness of grip. Loss of the normal distribution of forces at the wrist is the source of the pain, and reestablishing these relationships is the goal of treatment.

Lichtman stages range from 1 (diagnosis via magnetic resonance imaging or bone scan) to 4 (carpal collapse with osteoarthritis). Treatment ranges from radial reduction or ulnar lengthening to proximal row carpalectomy, although no consensus exists regarding effective treatment. Innervation can be seen in Figure 6.22.

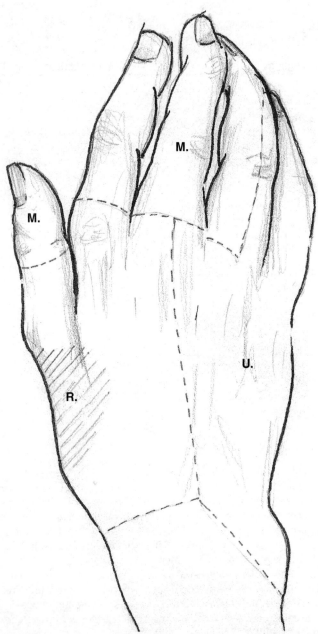

Figure 6.22 Hand dermatome. Note the areas supplied by the radial (R.), ulnar (U.), and median (M.) nerves.

Quick Look • Wrist and Hand

Inspect the skin, looking for gross deformity, guarding, or bruising.

Palpate the soft tissues surrounding the wrist and fingers. If infection is suspected, inspect for Kanavel signs.

Move wrist through ROM.
- Wrist flexion: 90°.
- Wrist extension: 75–90°.
- Radial deviation: 10–30°.
- Ulnar deviation: 10–30°.
- Move individual MCP, PIP, and DIP joints, noting pain or decreased ROM out of proportion to other digits.

Evaluate muscles using **special tests** to isolate the disorder.
- **Allen test:** Radial artery versus ulnar artery sufficiency. Ask patient to squeeze his or her hand several times, then hold a fist while occluding the radial and then the ulnar artery. Digital artery perfusion. Apply pressure to the lateral borders of the finger to the digital arteries.
- **Bunnel-Littler test:** Distinguishes between phalangeal intrinsic muscle tightness and joint capsule contracture. With some flexion, attempt to flex the PIP joint. Then, flex some at the MCP joint.
- **Differentiating flexor digitorum superficialis and flexor digitorum profundus:** Tendon or slip injury. Immobilize proximal joint, flex digit distally.
- **Finkelstein test:** Tenosynovitis. Patient makes a fist with the thumb tucked in and the hand tilted toward the little finger.
- **Froment test:** Ulnar neuropathy. Instruct the patient to pinch a piece of paper.
- **Opposition test:** Median neuropathy/opponens pollicis. Patient pinches using the thumb and little finger.
- **Phalen's sign:** Carpal tunnel syndrome. Bilateral volar wrist flexion for 30–60 seconds.
- **Pinch test:** Anterior interosseous neuropathy/weakness of flexor pollicis longus. Patient pinches with the thumb and index finger.
- **Regan test:** Lunotriquetral ligament tear. Stabilize lunate while manipulating ulnar aspect of wrist, feeling for instability.

- **Retinacular test:** Distinguishes between retinacular tightness and capsule contracture. Flex the DIP while holding the PIP.
- **Tinel's sign:** Carpal tunnel syndrome. Tap directly over the median nerve.
- **Watson test:** Scapholunate interosseus ligament tear. Palpate volar scaphoid. Dorsiflex and ulnar deviate the wrist, and then radially deviate volar wrist flex.

Reflex testing if neurologic deficits, cervical stenosis, or upper motor neuron (UMN)/lower motor neuron (LMN) disorder is suspected or if the patient is preoperative or postoperative.

- **Biceps (C5), brachioradialis (C6), triceps (C7).**
  - **Absent:** Neuropathy, LMN lesion.
  - **Hyperactive:** UMN lesion.

Order appropriate films.

- **PA:** Always assess DRUJ and carpal arcs/bones while assessing the digits. **All hand views should assess digit and metacarpal cortices, trabeculae, and articulations.**
  - Base of the thumb and fifth metacarpals (Bennett's, Rolando's, and boxer's fractures; gamekeeper's thumb).
  - Distal radius, DRUJ, ulnar styloid.
  - Scaphoid.
  - Metacarpal base, shaft, neck, and heads.
- **Lateral:** Check fractures at the interphalangeal joint.
- **Oblique (pronation):** The second and third metacarpals should be distinct.
- **Oblique (supination):** Compare hands, especially at the fifth digits.

SELECTED REFERENCES

Bonzar M, Firrell JC, Hainer M. Kienböck disease and negative ulnar variance. J Bone Joint Surg Am 1998 Aug;80(8):1154–1157.

Foster RJ, Hastings H II. Treatment of Bennett, Rolando, and vertical intra-articular trapezial fractures. Clin Orthop 1987 Jan;(214):121–129.

Hill N, Hurst L. Dupuytren's contracture. Hand Clin 1989;5:349–357.

Hueston JT, Wilson WF. The aetiology of trigger finger explained on the basis of intratendonous architecture. Hand 1972 Oct;4(3):257–260.

Kim J. Gamekeeper's thumb. Available at: http://www.emedicine.com/emerg/topic210.htm. Accessed April 13, 2006.

7

Hip

ANATOMY

Pelvis

The entire pelvis (Fig. 7.1) is actually a composite of the right and left hips, which in turn are comprised of three fused bones: the ilium, the ischium, and the pubis. Pelvic fusion begins at approximately 15 years of age and is complete by the mid-20s.

Ilium: This wing-shaped bone makes up the superior two-fifths of the acetabulum. Structurally, it is very important in load-bearing and muscular attachment. The anterior margin provides attachment for the iliopsoas and sartorius at the anterosuperior iliac spine. The anteroinferior iliac spine is the origin of the rectus femoris. The posteroinferior iliac spine is the superior margin of the greater sciatic notch, which transmits the sciatic nerve.

Ischium: The ischium contributes the posterior two-fifths of the acetabular cup. The ischial spine projects posteriorly and is the inferior point of the greater sciatic notch and the inferior point of the lesser sciatic notch. The ischial tuberosity is easily identified as the prominent bony projection that is felt when sitting down. The anteroinferior portion of the ischium is the ramus, which along with the pubic rami creates the oval obturator foramen.

Pubis: The pubis is the anterior fifth of the acetabulum and is comprised of roughly C-shaped superior and inferior pubic rami. It provides numerous muscular origins, including those of the pectineus, adductor longus, brevis, magnus, gracilis, obturator externus, and quadratus femoris. The pubic rami are common sites of fracture in trauma.

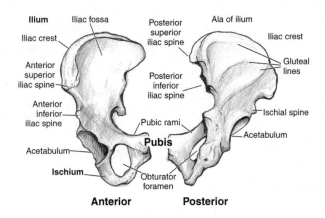

Ilium   Iliac fossa   Posterior   Ala of ilium
                              superior
Iliac crest   iliac spine   Iliac crest

Anterior   Gluteal
superior   Posterior   lines
iliac spine   inferior
                              iliac spine
Anterior
inferior   Ischial spine
iliac spine   Pubic rami
                          Pubis   Acetabulum
Acetabulum

Ischium   Obturator
                     foramen
        Anterior   **Posterior**

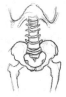

Figure 7.1 Bony pelvis.

Femur

The femur is so heavily invested with muscles that only the greater trochanter proximally and the femoral condyles distally are palpable.

Head: The ball-shaped femoral head sits tightly within the acetabular cup and is retained by a tough, fibrous capsule. The ligamentum capitis femoris enters the head in the center of the articular surface and, despite the presence of a small nutrient artery, receives most of its blood supply via the medial femoral circumflex artery. This blood supply enters the femoral neck and has tenuous distribution to the head, which makes the head prone to avascular necrosis when the medial femoral circumflex is disrupted.

Neck: The neck connects the body to the head at an angle of 125°. This structure ends at the intertrochanteric crest that runs between the greater trochanter superiorly and the lesser trochanter inferiorly.

Greater trochanter: The greater trochanter is important for the muscles that insert here, including the gluteus medius and minimus, piriformis, and obturator internus.

Lesser trochanter: This is the medial prominence at the junction of the body and neck, which can be avulsed in trauma because of its role as the insertion point for the powerful iliopsoas tendon.

Linea aspera: This is the rough, vertical ridge on the dorsal femur that provides insertion for the large adductors in addition to the three muscular septa that form the thigh compartments.

Muscular Anatomy and Motion

Tables 7.1 and 7.2 outline the basic muscular organization, function, and innervation of the pelvis, hip, and femur.

Vascular Anatomy and Neuroanatomy

Figures 7.2 and 7.3 show the anterior and posterior hemipelvis vascular and neuroanatomy.

BASIC EXAMINATION

Evaluation of the hip joint begins with the patient's gait as he or she walks into the examination room. Pain, limping, and muscular deficits are easily apparent, because they affect the patient's gait. Obvious traumatic deformities in the hip, which commonly present to the emergency department, should be memorized. The generalization to remember is shortened and internally rotated for hip dislocations and, as often is the case in elderly patients, shortened and externally rotated for a hip fracture. Dislocations are uncommon in the elderly, because bone usually gives way to force before it can dislocate. The Galeazzi test, or comparing leg length, is an easy way to rule out a basic anatomic disparity, whereas a Trendelenburg test can account for a gait disturbance that results from abductor weakness. Children can present with many abnormalities and should be evaluated for telescoping of the femur, leg-length discrepancies, joint laxity, and developmental dysplasia of the hip (DDH; formerly known as congenital hip dysplasia), which predisposes to hip dislocation. Flat feet (pes planus) are easily detected while examining gait. Hip pain in an obese, peripubescent child is a red flag for a slipped capitofemoral epiphysis (SCFE). The Ortolani and Barlow tests are the standards that should be performed in infants before they go home with the mother.

Inspection

Inspection begins with **gait** in the ambulatory patient and an exposed primary/secondary survey in the patient with trauma (Table 7.3).

Table 7.1 Muscles of the Hip

Muscle	Origin	Insertion
Gluteal		
Gluteus maximus	Ala of ilium, dorsal sacrum, and coccyx	Iliotibial band
Gluteus medius	Ilium	Lateral greater trochanter
Gluteus minimus	Ilium	Anterior greater trochanter
Piriformis	Anterior sacrum	Superior greater trochanter
Obturator internus	Pubic rami	Medial greater trochanter
Gemelli, superior and inferior	Superior ischial spine and inferior ischial tuberosity	Medial greater trochanter
Quadratus gemoris	Lateral ischial tuberosity	Intertrochanteric crest
Anterior thigh		
Psoas major	T12 through L5 vertebrae	Lesser trochanter via iliopsoas tendon
Iliacus	Iliac crest and fossa	Lesser trochanter via iliopsoas tendon
Tensor fascia lata	Anterosuperior iliac spine	Lateral tibial condyle
Sartorius	Anterosuperior iliac spine	Medial superior tibia
Rectus femoris	Anteroinferior iliac spine and superior acetabulum	Patella via quadriceps tendon
Vastus lateralis	Greater trochanter and lateral linea aspera	Patella via quadriceps tendon
Vastus medialis	Intertrochanteric line and medial linea aspera	Patella via quadriceps tendon
Vastus intermedius	Anterior and lateral body of femur	Patella via quadriceps tendon
Medial thigh		
Pectineus	Pubis (pectineal line)	Femur (pectineal line)

(continued on next page)

Table 7.1 Muscles of the Hip *(Continued)*

Muscle	Origin	Insertion
Adductor longus	Pubis (body)	Linea aspera (middle)
Adductor brevis	Pubis (body and inferior ramus)	Pectineal line and linea aspera (proximal)
Adductor magnus	Pubis (inferior ramus) and ischial tuberosity	Linea aspera and adductor tubercle
Gracilis	Pubis (body and inferior ramus)	Medial superior tibia
Obturator externus	Margin of obturator foramen	Trochanteric fossa
Posterior thigh		
Biceps femoris	Long head: Ischial tuberosity Short head: Lateral linea aspera	Lateral head of fibula (split by lateral collateral ligament)
Semimembranosus	Ischial tuberosity	Posterior medial tibial condyle
Semitendinosus	Ischial tuberosity	Medial superior tibia

Table 7.2 Muscular Motion of the Hip

Motion	Muscle	Innervation
Hip flexors		
Primary	Iliopsoas	Femoral nerve: L1, L2, and L3
Secondary	Rectus femoris	
Hip extensors		
Primary	Gluteus maximus	Inferior gluteal nerve: S1
Secondary	Hamstrings	
Abductors		
Primary	Gluteus medius	Superior gluteal nerve: L5
Secondary	Gluteus minimus	
Adductors		
Primary	Adductor longus	Obturator nerve: L2, L3, and L4
Secondary	Adductor brevis adductor and magnus pectineus gracilis	

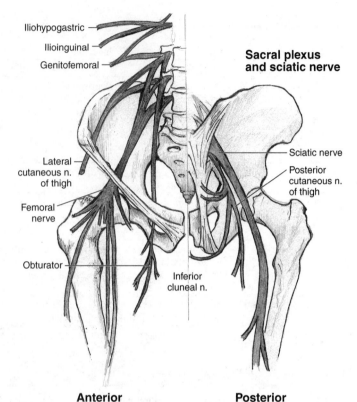

Anterior   **Posterior**

Figure 7.2 Sacral plexus and sciatic nerve. n., nerve.

- Heel-strike pain indicates a possible heel spur.
- Inability to decelerate before heel strike indicates weak hamstrings.

Deficits often relate to specific defects:

Deficit	Defect
Quadriceps weakness, back-knee gait, no toe-off, difficult to lock knee	L2 to L4
Tibialis anterior weakness, weak dorsiflexion, footdrop gait, steppage gait (high knee to keep foot from dragging)	L4
Gluteus medius, weakness on hip abduction, lateral lurch	L5

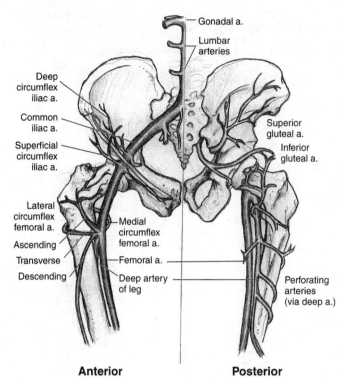

Figure 7.3 Vascular anatomy of the pelvis and proximal femur. a., artery.

| Gluteus maximus, weakness on hip extension, extensor lurch | S1 |
| Gastrocnemius/soleus weakness, flat-foot gait, no toe-off | S1 and S2 |

Observe the skin, and look for gross deformity, guarding, and bruising. In the supine patient, the legs should be equal in length and lie in slight external rotation. Hips should appear level and symmetric, and gluteal folds should be present and roughly even horizontally.

Palpation

Hips should be rocked and compressed, evaluating for tenderness, instability, or crepitus. Palpate the greater trochanter (trochanteric bursa). Pain at the anterosuperior iliac spine and characteristic football-shaped numbness on the lateral thigh can indicate meralgia paresthetica

Table 7.3 Etiology of Abnormal Gaits

Type	Description	Etiology
Propulsive gait	Weight centered forward with a stooped, rigid posture. The head and neck bent forward	Parkinson's disease Carbon monoxide poisoning Manganese poisoning Drugs, including antipsychotics
Scissors gait	Legs flexed slightly at the hips and knees, with the knees and thighs crossing in a scissors-like movement	Stroke Myelopathy Cervical spondylosis Advanced multiple sclerosis Spinal cord tumor Neurosyphilis/ meningomyelitis Syringomyelia Cerebral palsy Pernicious anemia/ vitamin B_{12} deficiency Liver failure
Spastic gait	Tonic unilateral muscular contraction. Upper extremity abducted and decorticate; lower extremity tonically extended and adducted	Brain tumor/trauma/ abscess Stroke Multiple sclerosis
Steppage gait	Footdrop with toes dragging on the ground while walking. Often compensates with a high-stepping gait and the foot slapping down	Guillain-Barré syndrome Multiple sclerosis Herniated lumbar disk Peroneal denervation/ atrophy Poliomyelitis Polyneuropathy Spinal cord trauma
Waddling gait	Distinctive, duck-like walk	Developmental dysplasia of the hip Muscular dystrophy Spinal muscle atrophy

via compression of the lateral femoral cutaneous nerve. Finally, palpate all muscle groups for symmetry.

The hips should be taken through a standard range-of-motion examination:

Abduction	40°
Adduction	30°
Flexion	130°
Hyperextension	20°
Internal rotation	30°
External rotation	50°

Note: Rotating the hips is unnecessary and potentially hazardous if there has been a previous arthroplasty. Check for normal rotation at the greater trochanteric angle (Fig. 7.4):

- **Increased retroversion:** Results in excessive external rotation and "toeing-out," limits internal rotation (e.g., **SCFE** in obese prepubescent and pubescent children).
- **Increased anteversion:** Results in excessive internal rotation and "toeing-in."

SPECIAL TESTS

Barlow Test

The Barlow test (Fig. 7.5) is used in infants and children to examine for congenital dislocation. Splay open the hips with your thumbs on the femurs and your fingers displacing the hip anteriorly. Feel for a dislocation click or **adduction** on the affected side. A positive test suggests DDH.

Digital Rectal Examination

This procedure is useful in orthopaedics for establishing the presence of coccygodynia. **Because of the appearance of the coccyx on radiographs, the digital rectal examination may provide the chief finding indicating fracture.**

Galeazzi Test

The Galeazzi test (Fig. 7.6) indicates femoral or tibial length discrepancy. In a supine patient with knees bent and feet on the table, evaluate the height of the knees.

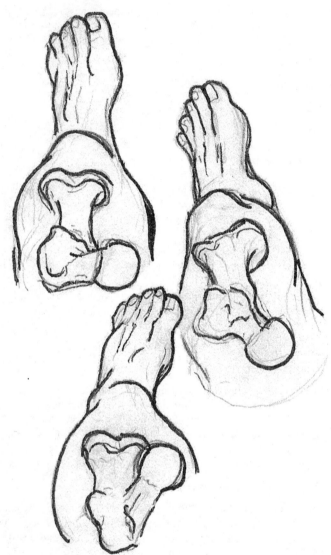

Figure 7.4 Trochanteric angle.

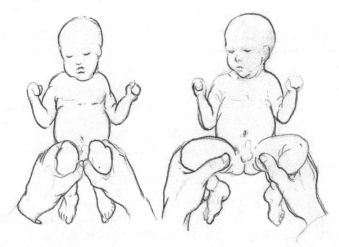

Figure 7.5 Barlow and Ortolani tests.

Ober Test

The Ober test is for the iliotibial band. When lying laterally, the patient flexes the knee 90° and abducts the leg. A positive result is the knee staying up when released, indicating a tight iliotibial band.

Ortolani Test

The Ortolani test (Fig. 7.5) is the same as the Barlow test, but **lack of abduction** causes dislocation. A positive test suggests DDH.

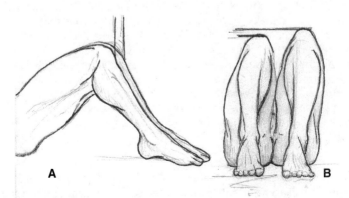

Figure 7.6 Galeazzi test: Femur length asymmetry and tibial length asymmetry.

Telescoping

Stabilize the hip and greater trochanter, and pull on the femur to feel for an inferior dislocation, similar to a sulcus sign in the humerus.

Thomas Test

The Thomas test is an examination for hip flexion contractures. In a supine patient, flex the knee and hip. A patient with flexion contractures cannot raise the knee to the chest without arching the lower back.

Note: Osteoarthritis limits motion in all planes, but especially internal rotation and abduction.

Trendelenburg Test

The Trendelenburg test (Fig. 7.7) involves a one-legged stance. Normally, the hip compensates superiorly; an inferior displacement of the hip means a weak abductor (gluteus medius).

RADIOLOGIC APPROACH TO THE PELVIS, HIP, AND FEMUR
Overview

Pelvic and hip fractures are a major source of morbidity and mortality in the elderly. Identification of fractures often is difficult. Such identification is essential, however, and requires multiple views. Femoral neck fractures endanger the blood supply to the hip via the circumflex arteries (anterior is most important). This creates a situation that may lead to avascular necrosis of the femoral head. The orientation of the trabecular pattern in the femoral neck is visible on plain-film radiographs and can provide clues to fractures that are difficult to image. These cases almost always require surgical reduction and fixation.

Computed tomography usually is ordered when pelvic fractures are suspected, because computed tomographic scans can allow better evaluation of these injuries. Many centers now offer three-dimensional reconstructions of the pelvis to evaluate complex pelvic fractures and plan operative management. The pelvis is a ring structure, and as such, a fracture almost always involves a compensating injury, such as another fracture in the ring or a disruption of the sacroiliac or pubic symphyseal ligaments.

Views

Note: Check to make sure you have the correct patient, the correct date, and the correct anatomy.

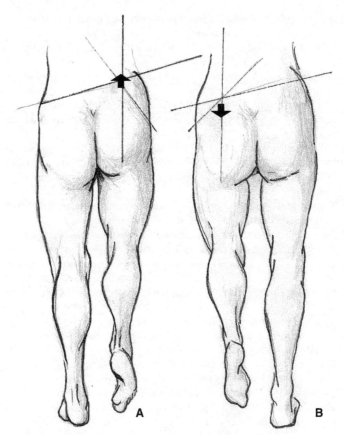

Figure 7.7 Trendelenburg test. A, Normal. B, Abnormal.

Anteroposterior View

The anteroposterior (AP) view may be the only practical view to obtain in a traumatic pelvic fracture, and the major classification systems use this view. An adequate view visualizes the entire pelvis and both hips. Although the pelvis should not be rotated, the femur should have approximately 15° of internal rotation to better expose the femoral neck. This causes the greater trochanter to be seen straight-on in profile, but the lesser trochanter is not as well depicted. This view of both hips is mandatory, but one hip also can be depicted individually so that the beam is centered on the neck (see Fig. 1.2, page 11). A line drawn along the femoral neck in an AP radiograph should intersect the lateral femoral-capital epiphysis; if not, it indicates SCFE, which can lead to avascular necrosis of the head.

When examining an AP view, be aware of the following guidelines:

- Overall, the hips, rami, sacroiliac joints, and acetabula should be symmetrical.
- The femoral head should be centered within the acetabulum with a normal, symmetric joint space averaging 4 mm superiorly and 8 mm medially.
- Follow the cortices of both femurs for continuity. This margin should be smooth except at the center of the femoral head (fovea centralis).
- Follow the pelvic cortex along both ala and around both the superior and inferior pubic rami.
- Tensile and compressive trabeculae should be scrutinized for disruption. Also scrutinize the intertrochanteric space.
- The Shenton's line should be intact and symmetric. Disruption of this interval often implies a neck fracture.
- The pubic symphysis should be in very close approximation. Distances of greater than 2.5 cm (diastasis) require surgical correction.
- Check the anterosuperior iliac spine, the anteroinferior iliac spine, and the greater and lesser trochanters for evidence of avulsion injuries (see origin and insertions above).
- Evaluate the radiologic teardrop of the anterior acetabular rim, acetabular surface, and ilioischial line.
- Evaluate the sacroiliac joints for symmetry and quality of margin. This can be a presenting site for ankylosing spondylitis.
- Evaluate the common areas of fracture in the acetabulum.
- The AP view of the pelvis provides a good depiction of the L5 transverse processes.

Frog-Leg View (Modified Cleaves)

Flexion at the knees, abduction, and external rotation of the hip provide a view that is perpendicular to the AP view. This frog-leg view (Fig. 7.8) provides a good depiction of the femoral neck and proximal femur, and it is essential for evaluating SCFE in children.

The **Klein's line** is a radiologic examination for pain in external rotation and flexion, usually in obese peripubescent children (median age, 12 years).

Cross-Table Lateral View

This view is shot with one leg elevated out of view and the beam directed at the medial groin superiorly across the hip and perpendicular to the femoral neck. Proximal femoral and acetabular fractures are depicted.

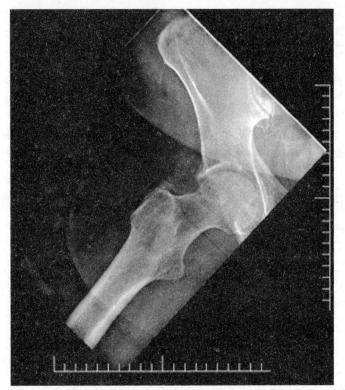

Figure 7.8 Frog-leg radiograph of the hip.

Anterior Oblique/Posterior Oblique Views

These views are used to depict the anterior and posterior columns as well as the acetabulum.

Internal/External Oblique (JUDET) Views

These trauma views are the indicated for the initial evaluation and intraoperative management of hip and **acetabular** fractures. The anterior and posterior columns and the acetabular rims are well depicted in this projection.

Inlet/Outlet Views

These views are used in evaluation of the pelvic rim and acetabulum for fractures. Sacroiliac joint separation can been seen in the inlet view, which uses a beam directly 45° caudally. The outlet view is shot in a cephalad direction and can better depict fractures of the sacrum, sacroiliac separation, and fractures of the anterior pubis.

SELECTED FRACTURES OF THE PELVIS, HIP, AND FEMUR

Hip Fracture

There are three main types of proximal femoral (hip) fractures: femoral neck, intertrochanteric, and subtrochanteric. Most often, these are associated with aging bones, underlying pathology (osteoporosis, cancer, or hypoparathyroidism), and trauma. Eighty percent of hip fractures occur in patients older than 60 years. Signs and symptoms of a hip fracture begin with an account of the mechanism of injury (e.g., a fall in the elderly or a dashboard injury in motor-vehicle accident). Pain ranging from mild in a nondisplaced fracture to severe in more significant fractures is present in the hip or groin or is transferred to the leg and knee. External rotation and shortening of the affected extremity is a classic sign but is not necessary. Plain-film radiography (AP and frog-leg lateral views), magnetic resonance imaging, and bone scan are sensitive for fracture, although radiography may not reveal fine, nondisplaced fractures. The pelvis, knees, and ankles should be thoroughly evaluated when a hip fracture is suspected.

Femoral neck fractures usually are seen with high-energy trauma in younger patients, generally in association with multiple injuries. High rates of avascular necrosis and nonunion are seen in this population. Outcome in this group can be roughly predicted by the extent, amount of displacement, comminuted areas, and disruption of vascular supply in addition to the success achieved with reduction and fixation (Fig. 7.9).

A significant portion (10–15%) of patients have poor results despite good orthopaedic care, mostly as a result of vascular compromise and eventual avascular necrosis. The vascular supply to the femoral neck is notoriously bad to begin with, and it has little or no periosteum, which is where the majority of bone healing takes place. Nonunion rates for these fractures are high, which necessitates urgent, gentle reduction and fixation.

Although many different devices are used for internal fixation of femoral neck fractures, two are most common: multiple cannulated screws and compression screws/metal plate combinations, often with an antirotation screw. Good success usually is obtained with fixation using cannulated screws.

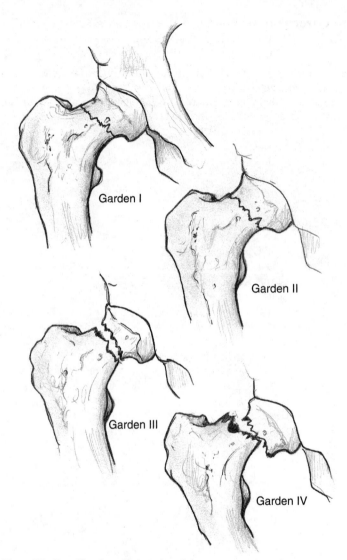

Figure 7.9 Classification of femoral neck fracture.

Intertrochanteric Fractures

There are four types of intertrochanteric fractures (Fig. 7.10):

- **Type I:** Extend along the intertrochanteric line from the greater to the lesser trochanter.
- **Type II:** Comminuted fractures, again extending along the main intertrochanteric line.

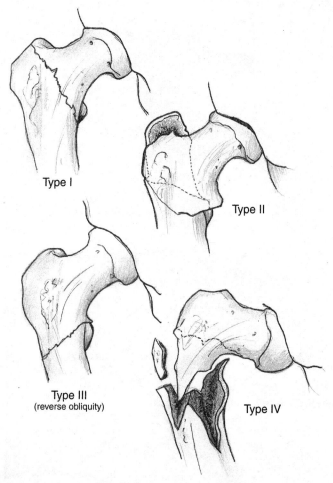

Figure 7.10 Intertrochanteric fractures: Boyd and Griffin classification.

- **Type III:** Basically subtrochanteric fractures, with at least one fracture near or at the lesser trochanter.
- **Type IV:** In the trochanteric region and the proximal shaft, with fracture in at least two planes. Many methods can be used for operative fixation of an intertrochanteric fracture, ranging from reconstruction nails and plates with cannulated screws to total hip replacement using a metal implant.

Subtrochanteric Fractures

Subtrochanteric fractures often are associated with high-energy trauma, such as motor-vehicle accidents in the young, and with low-velocity trauma, such as falls in the elderly. Intertrochanteric fractures often require open reduction and internal fixation. Subtrochanteric fractures can be classified by the Russell-Taylor criteria as either type I (piriformis fossa intact) or type II (fractured) and subclassified as type A (lesser trochanter intact) or type B (less trochanter fractured) (Figs. 7.11 and 7.12). Today, treatment often involves the use of an intramedullary reconstruction nail.

SELECTED DISORDERS OF THE PELVIS, HIP, AND FEMUR
Developmental Dysplasia of the Hip

Although many theories exist for the etiology of DDH, the consensus is that it is a multifactorial disorder, with both intrauterine and extrauterine factors as well as congenital and mechanical influences. The incidence is sixfold greater in girls than in boys at birth, where it often is picked up by orthopaedic screening using the Ortolani and Barlow tests. Whatever the etiology, however, the outcome is an easily dislocating hip within the acetabulum. If this is not detected either at or shortly after birth, it leads to secondary femoral and acetabular changes in the adolescent, who is permanently disabled. In a child who has matured somewhat with a nonreducible dislocation, the assessment includes the following three factors: decreased hip abduction because of adductor contracture; asymmetrical inguinal, popliteal, and gluteal skin folds; and apparent shortening of the affected leg (positive Galeazzi test). A waddling gait may be reported in an older child who has matured with a dislocated hip.

Treatment of the newborn involves extended use of a traction device (Pavlik harness), which helps reduce the dislocation and prevent serious adductor contractures. This treatment has a high degree of success in newborns and select infants, but it does not work in older patients. These older patients require individual surgical correction, which may involve reduction, tenotomy, arthrography, and pelvic

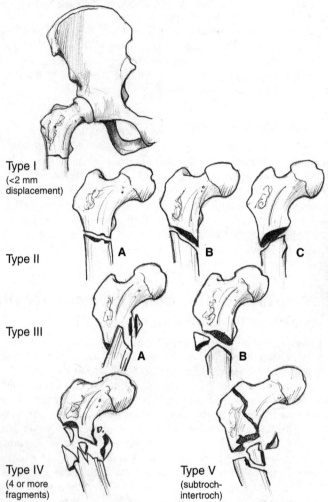

Type I
(<2 mm
displacement)

Type II   A   B   C

Type III   A   B

Type IV
(4 or more
fragments)

Type V
(subtroch-
intertroch)

Figure 7.11 Subtrochanteric fractures: Seinsheimer classification.

osteotomy, with various methods of postsurgical cast or spica immobilization. Success rates with these advanced procedures are variable.

Slipped Capitofemoral Epiphysis

Slipped capitofemoral epiphysis is the most common orthopaedic disorder of the adolescent hip. Seen most typically in peripubescent

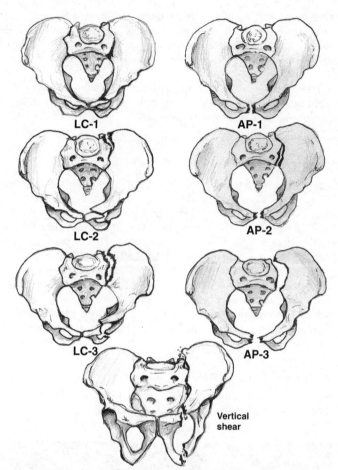

Figure 7.12 Young and Burgess classification of pelvic ring fractures.

obese males (although it occurs in females as well), it can present as a variable cluster of hip thigh and knee pain. It is commonly missed (30–50% of cases), because it frequently appears in the absence of trauma and can be subtle on radiographs if it is not the specific object of investigation. Young patients may complain of a preceding pop or a gradual progression from a dull ache to a pain when ascending stairs. Internal rotation, abduction, and flexion are reduced, and external rotation that occurs with hip flexion is a key sign and is considered to be almost pathognomonic. The preferred radiographic views are the AP and the frog-leg lateral, which is the most sensitive. In the AP view,

Klein's line describes a line drawn along the superior femoral neck, which should intersect the femoral head; if it does not, an SCFE should be suspected. In the frog-leg lateral view, a widening and blurring of the physis (Bloomberg's sign) also is diagnostic of SCFE and, in a subtle case, may be the only sign.

Treatment, which usually involves screw fixation, is essential to prevent deformity and disability. Failure to treat can lead to healing of the dislocation in an anatomically poor position and to early osteoarthritis and even avascular necrosis.

Unicameral Bone Cyst

Figure 7.13 shows a unicameral bone cyst. These lesions are not true neoplasms and are found predominantly in children within the first two decades of life. These radiolucent areas are like other cysts (i.e., fluid-filled cavities lined by fibrous tissue) and usually are found in the metaphysis of long bones. Radiographically, these cysts generally respect the cortices and do not contain fluid levels. They are considered to be benign, and they cause no symptoms unless they lead to a pathological fracture. If found incidentally at radiography and not disrupting an active growth plate, treatment is conservative, and the cyst should be followed to watch for growth. If a fracture occurs, treatment can involve curettage and bone grafting. Other treatments are injection of steroids or bone marrow.

Aneurysmal Bone Cysts

Figure 7.14 shows an aneurysmal bone cyst. In contrast to simple unicameral cysts, aneurysmal bone cysts are painful and may be palpa-

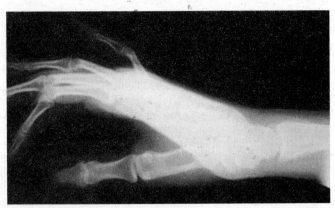

Figure 7.13 Radiograph of a unicameral bone cyst.

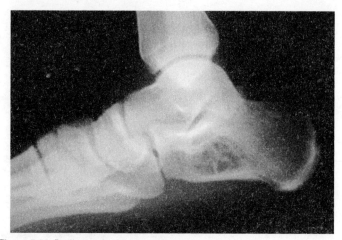

Figure 7.14 Radiograph of an aneurysmal bone cyst.

ble. These cysts can arise as the primary disorder from an unknown cause, or they can occur secondarily from another tumor, such as a chondroblastoma, osteosarcoma, or giant cell tumor of bone. The spine, metaphysis of the femur, and proximal tibia are common sites. Treatment is essentially the same as for simple bone cysts, although the vascular extent of these tumors needs to be assessed before surgery to avoid excessive blood loss. Radiographically, these cysts often bow the cortices and expand the intramedullary canal.

Subchondral Cysts

Subchondral cysts often are secondary to degenerative joint disease following eburnation of bone as a result of joint compression. They are found just superficial to the articular surface of the joint and surrounded by a dense rim of sclerotic bone. All types of bone cysts are rather easily identified on radiographs as radiolucent areas.

Avascular Necrosis

Necrosis implies dead, infracted bone resulting from a number of pathological conditions. Common predisposing conditions include femoral neck fractures in the elderly, sickle cell disease, systemic lupus erythematosus (because of chronic corticosteroid use), or Legg-Calvé-Perthes disease, which can be diffuse to the femoral head. Avascular necrosis shows as increased density on magnetic resonance images.

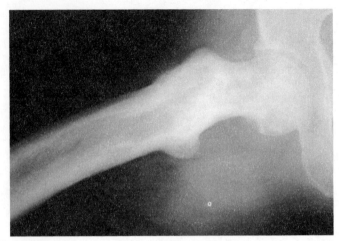

Figure 7.15 Radiograph of a hip with Paget's disease.

Paget's Disease

Figure 7.15 shows a hip with Paget's disease. This pathological resorption of bone results from alternating phases of uncontrolled osteoclastic resorption and osteoblastic formation. It results in a "mosaic" bone that lacks the normal lamellar structure, which can lead to arteriovenous fistulas (potential for high-output heart failure), enlargement of the cranium, deafness, bone pain, and increased risk of osteogenic sarcoma. Orthopaedic surgery in this patient population is risky and needs to be planned with care, because bleeding can be very significant. Increased osteocalcin and pyridinium urinary collagen cross-links are seen on specific urinalysis.

Quick Look • **Hip**

Inspect the skin, looking for gross deformity, guarding, and bruising. Hips should appear level and symmetric, with even gluteal folds.

Palpate the hips, which should be rocked and compressed to evaluate for tenderness, instability, or crepitus. Palpate the greater trochanter (trochanteric bursa).

Move the hips through flexion and hyperextension, adduction, abduction, and internal and external rotation. Rotating the hips is unnecessary and potentially hazardous in patients with a previous arthroplasty.

- **Abduction:** 40°.
- **Adduction:** 30°.
- **Flexion:** 130°.
- **Hyperextension:** 20°.
- **Internal rotation:** 30°.
- **External rotation:** 50°.

Evaluate muscles using **special tests** to isolate the disorder.

- **Barlow test:** Same as the Ortolani test, but **adduction** causes dislocation; DDH.
- **Digital rectal examination:** Coccygodynia.
- **Galeazzi test:** Femoral or tibial length discrepancy in a supine patient; knees bent and feet on table; evaluate height of knees.
- **Ober test:** Iliotibial band contractures; patient lying lateral; flex knee 90°, and abduct leg.
- **Ortolani test:** Splay open hips with thumbs on femurs and fingers displacing hip anteriorly; dislocation click or lack of **abduction** on the affected side; DDH.
- **Telescoping:** Stabilize hip and greater trochanter; pull femur to feel for an inferior dislocation.
- **Thomas test:** Hip flexion contractures; flex knee and hip in a supine patient.
- **Trendelenburg test:** Weak abductor (gluteus medius); one-legged stance.

Order appropriate radiographic views.

- **Anteroposterior:**
  - Overall, the hips, rami, sacroiliac joints, and acetabulum should be symmetric.
  - Femoral head centered within the acetabulum; normal, symmetric joint space.
  - Intact cortices of both femurs, hip, and pelvis.
  - Scrutinize tensile and compressive trabeculae for disruption.
  - Shenton's line intact, symmetric.
  - Pubic symphysis in close approximation (diastasis, >2.5 cm).
  - Check the anterosuperior iliac spine, anteroinferior iliac spine, and greater and lesser trochanters for evidence of avulsion injuries.

- – Evaluate the radiologic teardrop, acetabular surface, and ilioischial line.
- – Sacroiliac joints symmetric.
- – Evaluate the common areas of fracture in the acetabulum.
- – Intact L5 transverse processes.
- **Frog leg:** Perpendicular to the AP view; evaluate for SCFE in children.
- **Cross-table lateral:** Check for proximal femoral and acetabular fractures.
- **Anterior oblique/posterior oblique:** Intact anterior and posterior columns as well as the acetabulum.
- **Internal/external oblique (JUDET):** Evaluation and intraoperative management of hip and acetabular fractures; intact anterior/posterior columns and acetabulum.
- **Inlet/outlet:** Evaluate the pelvic rim and acetabulum for fractures; rule out sacroiliac joint separation, fractures of the sacrum, and anterior pubic fractures.

Reflex testing if neurologic deficits, cervical stenosis, or upper motor neuron (UMN)/lower motor neuron (LMN) disorder is suspected or if the patient is preoperative or postoperative.

- **Patellar (L4), Achilles (S1).**
  - **Absent:** Neuropathy, LMN lesion.
  - **Hyperactive:** UMN lesion.

SELECTED REFERENCES

Bancroft LW, Peterson JJ, Kransdorf MJ. Cysts, geodes, and erosions. Radiol Clin North Am 2004;42:73–87.

Canale ST. Campbell's Operative Orthopaedics. 10th ed. Philadelphia: Mosby, 2003:796–799.

Hullar TE. Paget's disease and fibrous dysplasia. Otolaryngol Clin North Am 2003;36:707–732.

Perron AD, Miller MD, Brady WJ. Orthopaedic pitfalls in the ED: slipped capital femoral epiphysis. Am J Emerg Med 2002;20: 484–487.

Reynolds RAK. Diagnosis and treatment of slipped capital femoral epiphysis. Curr Opin Pediatr 1999;11:80–83.

Schneider D. Diagnosis and treatment of Paget's disease of bone. Am Fam Physician 2002;65:2069–2072.

8

Knee

The knee is illustrated in Figure 8.1.

ANATOMY

Bony and Ligamentous Anatomy

The knee is a hinge-type joint that is capable of significant flexion but limited extension and rotation. It is a large synovial joint with a thin, fibrous capsule that contains synovium and is in contact with the femoral condyles, patella, and tibia. The medial and lateral aspects of the joint receive additional support from the medial and lateral collateral ligaments, iliotibial band, and pes anserinus.

Other parts of the knee include:

Distal femur: Two large femoral condyles span the articular surface, separated by a large groove called the intercondylar notch. The notch glides under the articular surface of the patella and also gives space for the cruciate ligaments. The medial supracondylar ridge gives insertion to several muscles, as does the adductor tubercle, which also is medial, just above the condyles.

Patella: This is the largest sesamoid bone (developed within a tendon) in the body. The patella is believed to act either by increasing the mechanical advantage of the quadriceps or by reducing friction on the tendons over the intercondylar notch. It is not uncommon to find bipartite patella (a patella that failed to fuse during the first 6 years of life).

Tibia: This large, weight-bearing bone is commonly fractured; in fact, it may be the most commonly fractured bone. The tibial plateau articulates with the femoral condyles, and when loaded, the articular cartilage of the femur and tibia glide across each other. Osteoarthritis of the knee is very common and occurs when this cartilage wears down. The vascular supply to the tibia is tenuous and may result in long healing times

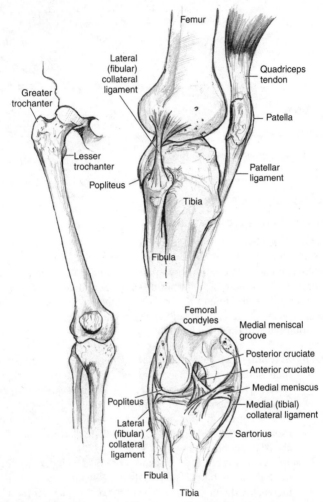

Figure 8.1 Dermatome of umbilicus to popliteal fossa.

and nonunion for the fractured bone. Anteriorly, the tibial tuberosity accepts the patellar tendon. Medially, the semi-membranosus and popliteus insert.

Fibula: This bone has no weight-bearing role; however, it does serve a role in stabilizing the tibia and providing attachment for muscles. The lateral collateral (fibular collateral) ligament connects the lateral femoral condyle to the fibula. The common fibular (peroneal) nerve courses around the fibular head and is vulnerable to injury here.

Menisci: There are two C-shaped cartilaginous menisci, medial and lateral. Their chief role is filling the gap between the femoral condyles and the tibial plateau. Other roles include cushioning and distributing applied vertical load and facilitating smooth movement while adding structural support for even wear of the articular cartilage. The menisci lie within the joint capsule but outside the synovial capsule. When torn, they present as obstacles to smooth tracking of the knee, often catching in the joint space and giving characteristic symptoms of locking, popping, and limited motion. The main difference between the two menisci is the attachment of the medial meniscus to the medial collateral ligament. This predisposes it to tearing more often because of its lack of free motion when caught between opposing forces (e.g., twisting the knee while bent). Like all tough cartilage, the menisci are largely avascular; therefore, healing a meniscal injury is very difficult.

Transverse ligament: Both menisci insert into the anterior intercondylar area of the tibia and are spanned by the transverse ligament.

Posterior meniscofemoral ligament: This strong, tendinous connection joins the lateral meniscus to the posterior cruciate ligament at the medial femoral condyle.

Cruciate ligaments:

- **Anterior cruciate ligament (ACL):** The distinctions between the anterior and posterior cruciate ligaments are in function. The ACL prevents excessive forward translation of the tibia relative to the femur, and it limits the knee in hyperextension. When the knee is flexed, however, the ACL serves no role and is lax. The ACL derives it name from its attachment to the anterior intercondylar area of the tibial eminence.

- **Posterior cruciate ligament (PCL):** The role of the PCL is complementary to the ACL. It prevents excessive rearward translation of the tibia in flexion, limiting hyperflexion of the knee. Because this is a difficult position in which to sustain an injury, a characteristic mechanism often is present (e.g., striking the dashboard with the knee in a motor-vehicle accident, driving the tibial backward while the body is thrust forward).

Collateral ligaments:

- **Medial (tibial) collateral ligament (MCL):** This ligament limits the lateral motion of the knee and abduction of the leg at the knee. The bulk of support in all directions of the knee, however, comes from the joint spanning musculature provided by the quadriceps, adductors, iliotibial band, and gastrocnemius–soleus groups. Injury to the MCL often entails damage to the medial meniscus, which is invested in the ligament. Sudden force directed at the lateral knee (e.g., spearing in football or an automobile bumper vs. pedestrian accident) can disrupt the MCL, medial meniscus, and ACL, resulting in the so-called "unhappy triad." The MCL, as opposed to the LCL, is a broader, fibrous band, whereas the LCL is a rounded cord.

- **Lateral collateral ligament (LCL):** This ligament limits the knee from excessive varus angulation. It has an origin at the superior lateral femoral condyle, and it inserts on the fibular head.

Figure 8.2 illustrates the anterior knee, and Figure 8.3 illustrates of the lateral knee.

Muscular Anatomy

Tables 8.1 and 8.2 outline the basic muscular organization and innervation found in the knee (see Fig. 8.3).

Vascular and Neuroanatomy

Figure 8.4 shows the course of the common fibular nerve and the anterior tibial nerve.

BASIC EXAMINATION

A complete assessment of the knee is the bread and butter of orthopaedics. The patient history and physical examination findings are key, and the radiologic findings should only be supportive of the examination. Pain and the mechanism of injury are important findings and can help in establishing the diagnosis. For instance, ACL injuries are associated with cutting movements and can have a "pop" associated with the injury. Injuries to the PCL are infrequent but factor large in the evaluation of dashboard injuries. Injuries that involve twisting and subsequent locking of the knee suggest meniscal injuries. Locking also can be a sign of loose bodies in the joint space. Degenerative joint diseases, in contrast, appear in the absence of trauma, are chronic in nature, and have a reliable pattern of pain or disability. A complaint of swelling can suggest fractures and ligamentous injuries in the acute

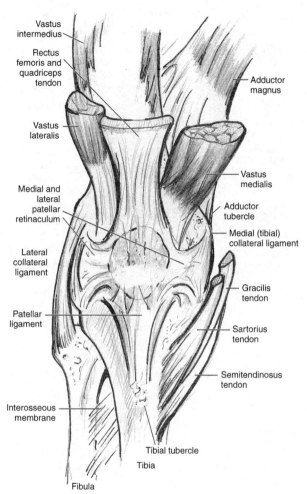

Figure 8.2 Anterior knee.

setting, whereas meniscal and chondral injuries have delayed swelling. A medial (or lateral) knee effusion associated with a subpatellar grinding suggests patellofemoral pain.

Observation

The examination should start with observation (Table 8.3). Whether a knee is varus or valgus, which predisposes to injury and pathology,

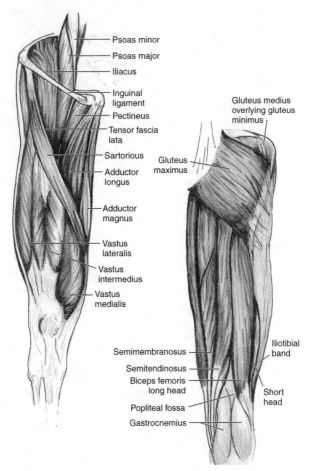

Figure 8.3 Lateral knee.

should be noted, and muscular atrophy should not be missed. Gait disturbances factor in a large number of knee and other problems. Table 8.4 outlines some conditions that should be considered in the differential diagnosis of the knee.

Palpation

Palpate the knee, looking for signs of effusion. The ballottement test and bulge sign should be performed, milking the superior part of the

Table 8.1 Muscles of the Knee

	Origin	Insertion
Knee flexion		
Semimembranosus	Ischial tuberosity	Posterior medial tibial condyle
Semitendinosus	Ischial tuberosity	Medial superior tibia
Biceps femoris	Long head: Ischial tuberosity Short head: Lateral linea aspera	Lateral head of fibula (split by lateral collateral ligament)
Gracilis	Pubis (body and inferior ramus)	Medial superior tibia
Sartorius	Anterior superior iliac spine (ASIS)	Medial superior tibia
Popliteus	Lateral condyle	Posterior tibia
Knee extension		
Rectus femoris	1. Anterior inferior iliac spine 2. Superior acetabulum	Patella via quadriceps tendon
Vastus lateralis	Greater trochanter lateral linea aspera	Patella via quadriceps tendon
Vastus intermedius	Anterior and lateral body of femur	Patella via quadriceps tendon
Vastus medialis	Intertrochanteric line and medial linea aspera	Patella via quadriceps tendon
Tensor fascia lata	ASIS	Lateral tibial condyle
Medial tibial rotation		
Popliteus	Lateral condyle	Posterior tibia
Semimembranosus	Ischial tuberosity	Posterior medial tibial condyle
Semitendinosus	Ischial tuberosity	Medial superior tibia
Sartorius	ASIS	Medial superior tibia
Gracilis	Pubis (body and inferior ramus)	Medial superior tibia
Lateral tibial rotation		
Biceps femoris	Long head: Ischial tuberosity Short head: Lateral linea aspera	Lateral head of fibula (split by lateral collateral ligament)

Table 8.2 Muscle Groups of the Knee and Their Innervation

Muscles	Muscle Group	Nerve (Root)
Extension	Quadriceps	Femoral nerve (L2, L3, and L4)
Flexion	Hamstrings	Tibial portion of sciatic nerve (L5)

patella if necessary. The patella should move freely but not excessively, as in a patient who is prone to dislocation (an apprehension test can help detect a dislocator).

Range of Motion

Move the knee through its normal range of motion:

Flexion	135°
Extension	0–5°
Internal rotation	10°
External rotation	10°

Check squat and extension. Difficulty in the last 10° of extension indicates quadriceps weakness.

Abnormal knee alignments:

- **Genu varum:** Bowed legs.
- **Genu valgum:** Knock knees.
- **Genu recurvatum:** Back knees.

Reflex

The patellar reflex involves tapping the patellar tendon with a hammer.

SPECIAL TESTS

Anterior Drawer Test

The anterior drawer test indicates ACL insufficiency (see *Lachman Test* below). Pull the tibia forward and away from femur in a 90° flexed knee; a normal knee should not have significant tibial travel.

Apley Test

The Apley test (Fig. 8.5) is for medial and lateral meniscal tears. The patient lies prone, with the knee flexed. Press down on the heel, and rotate the tibia. A positive test is pain on the side of the tear.

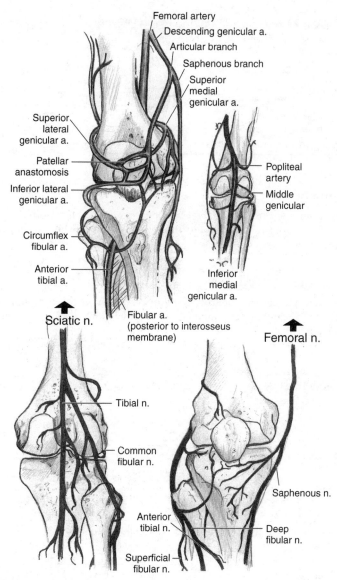

Figure 8.4 Course of common fibular nerve and anterior tibial nerve. a., artery; n., nerve.

Table 8.3 Role of Examination in the Diagnosis of Knee Disorders

Observation	Problem
Antalgic gait	Pain in affected leg
Trendelenburg sign	Weak hip abductors
Medial or lateral thrust of affected knee	Posterolateral or posteromedial injury
Squatting pain	Meniscal tear

Apprehension Test

The apprehension test indicates dislocation and subluxation of the patella. Try to laterally dislocate the patella. A patient who is prone to dislocation reacts with anxiety/pain.

Ballottement Test

Push the patella into the trochlear groove. A positive test is rebounding of the patella from a fluid-filled joint, indicating significant knee effusion.

Table 8.4 Differential Diagnosis of Knee Pathology

	Age (years)	Sex	Onset	Joint Stiffness	Deformity
Meniscal tear	15–60	Male	Sudden with sports	Locking	Swelling
Osteoarthritis	50–80	Female	Gradual	Yes (AM)	Flexion contractures
Rheumatoid arthritis	5–80+	Female	Gradual	Yes (AM and PM)	Flexion contractures
Anterior cruciate ligament injury	25–55	Male	Sudden with sports	"Giving out"	Recurvatum with posterior cruciate ligament tear

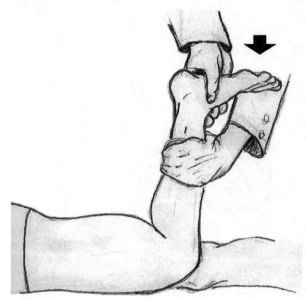

Figure 8.5 Apley test.

Bounce Home Test

Flex the knee in an elevated leg, which should fall straight. If not, this suggests swelling in a joint.

Bulge Sign

Press the lateral aspect of the knee, and observe for a medial knee bulge (Fig. 8.6), indicating a minor knee effusion.

Distraction Test

The distraction test is similar to the Apley test, but it distinguishes between meniscal and ligamentous damage. The test involves pulling upward traction as opposed to downward compression. Pain suggests damage to the ligament, not a torn menisci.

External Rotation Recurvatum Test

The external rotation recurvatum test (Fig. 8.7) assesses for PCL insufficiency. Pick up the extended leg by the foot. A positive test is the knee going into the varus position and recurvatum.

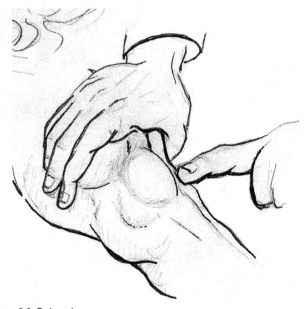

Figure 8.6 Bulge sign.

Lachman Test

The Lachman test (Fig. 8.8) indicates ACL insufficiency. Pull the tibia forward and away from the femur in a 30° flexed knee; a normal knee should not have significant tibial travel.

Note: A positive Lachman may be the only observable sign in a traumatic knee.

McMurray Test

The McMurray test (Fig. 8.9) was developed to assess posterior meniscal tears. Apply valgus stress while externally rotating the bent knee in a supine patient. A positive test is a painful click, indicating meniscal instability.

Note: A reduction click occurs when a McMurray test unlocks a locked knee.

Pivot Shift Test

The pivot shift test (Fig. 8.10) indicates ACL insufficiency. Place valgus stress at the knee joint, with some internal rotation, while moving

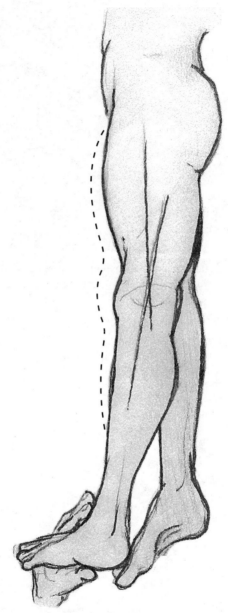

Figure 8.7 External rotation recurvatum test.

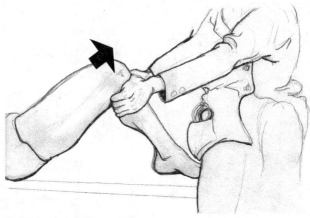

Figure 8.8 Lachman test.

the knee though flexion at the knee joint. A normal knee should move smoothly. A positive test is a clunky pivot during flexion.

Posterior Drawer Test

This test indicates PCL insufficiency (see *Lachman Test* above). Push the tibia backward and away from the femur in a 90° flexed knee; a normal knee should not have significant tibial travel. Also try the quadriceps active test.

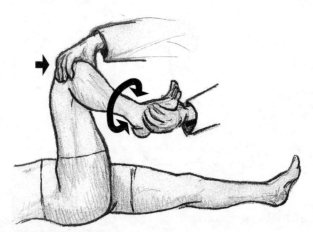

Figure 8.9 McMurray test.

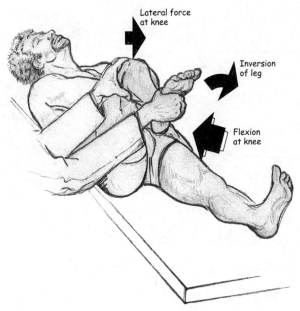

Figure 8.10 Pivot shift test.

Quadriceps Active Test

The quadriceps active test (Fig. 8.11) indicates PCL tear. With the patient's knee at approximately 80°, apply posterior stress on the tibia at the ankle joint, and instruct the patient to resist motion by firing the quadriceps (extending the leg, but resisted). A positive test is anterior translation of the tibia.

Varus/Valgus Test

The varus/valgus test (Fig. 8.12) assesses collateral ligaments. In a 30° flexed knee, stress is applied in varus and valgus to assess collateral laxity. Positive varus laxity is an LCL weakness/tear, and positive valgus laxity is an MCL weakness/tear.

RADIOLOGIC APPROACH TO THE KNEE
Overview

Many knee injuries involve soft tissue and ligamentous injuries, but with no observable signs on radiographs. One of the first considerations for obtaining knee radiographs is determining which patients

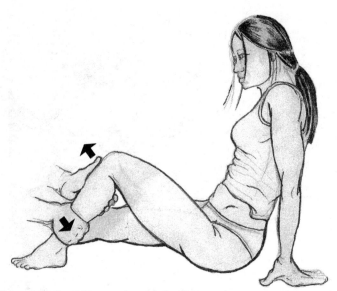

Figure 8.11 Quadriceps active test. Feel for anterior movement.

need them. A great deal of research in emergency medicine concerns who benefits. Some of these criteria include:

Elderly (>55 years)
Tenderness of fibular head
Knee effusion
Significant bruising
Isolated patellar tenderness
Knee flexion <90°
Nonweight bearing
Pain with a previous knee replacement

For diagnosed fractures, use of computed tomography (CT) often is of benefit, especially in cases of tibial plateau fractures. Three-dimensional reconstruction is an excellent tool for imaging complex fractures. Magnetic resonance imaging (MRI), on the other hand, is much better for detecting soft tissue injuries. Meniscal tears, ACL/PCL damage, and avulsion injuries are best depicted by MRI.

Views

Note: Check to make sure you have the correct patient, the correct date, and the correct anatomy.

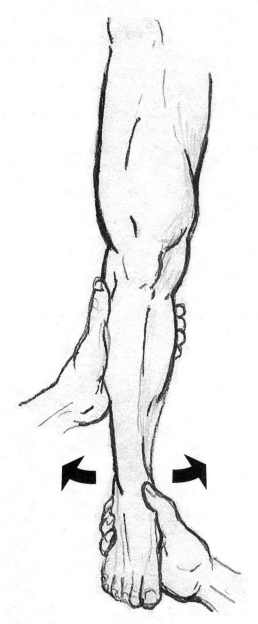

Figure 8.12 Varus/valgus test.

Anteroposterior View

In the adequate anteroposterior (AP) radiograph (Fig. 8.13) of the knee, the tibial spines (intercondylar eminences) are centered between the femoral condyles. The femoral condyles are not rotated, with equal medial and lateral joint spaces. The patella is midline and just superior to the joint space.

Because the area of most disability (and liability) is the tibial plateau, it should be the focus of the initial survey:

- Follow the tibial cortex through all visible margins.
- Scrutinize the trabeculae for any evidence of fracture, impaction, or unexplained densities.
- Articular surfaces are of obvious importance, and fracture fragments can be small.
- The supracondylar femur is another disabling fracture and should be sought.
- The margin of the patella can be examined under hot light. The image of the patella is superimposed on the distal femur, and subtle fractures of the patella are difficult to detect.

The normal variants of the patella must be kept in mind, because a failure of the developing patella ossification centers to fuse can be mistaken for a fracture.

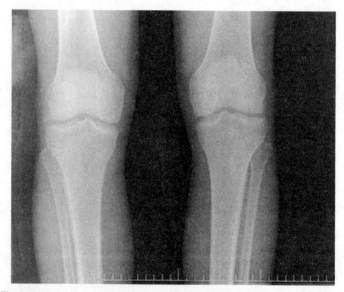

Figure 8.13 Anteroposterior radiograph of the knee.

Lateral View

A good lateral radiograph (Fig. 8.14) should not be rotated, and the femoral condyles will be in line with nearly complete overlap. The fibula is separate, and the AP margins of the tibia and fibula are distinct. The patella sits anterior to the joint space.

When examining a lateral radiograph, keep the following in mind:

- This view is evaluated in the same way as the AP view, with the two views giving a full survey of the tibial plateau.
- Despite the overlap of the femoral condyles, this view gives good visualization of the AP condyles.

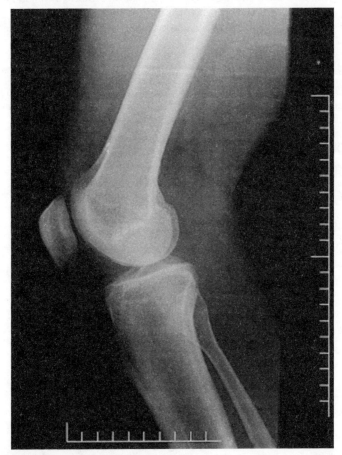

Figure 8.14 Lateral radiograph of the knee.

Table 8.5 Lateral Knee and Insall-Salvati Ratio[a]

	Patella Baja	Patella Alta
Insall-Salvati ratio	<0.8	>1.2
Cause	Quadriceps tendon rupture Achondroplasia	Patellar tendon rupture

[a]Measure from the tibial tuberosity to the inferior patella, and divide by the length of the patella in 30° of flexion.

- Evaluate the patella using the Insall-Salvati ratio (infrapatellar length/patella length) (Table 8.5).
- Fat/blood levels are always a clue to the presence of an intra-articular fracture.

Sunrise (Merchant) View

The sunrise (Merchant) view (Fig. 8.15) is commonly used by joint replacement specialists, because it shows how the patella sits in the intercondylar groove. Vertical patellar fractures also are visible.

Oblique View

Because of the importance of noting fractures of the femoral condyles and tibial plateau, this view is included in the standard knee series (see *Tibial Plateau Fractures* below).

SELECTED FRACTURES OF THE KNEE

Ottawa Knee Rules

Salter-Harris classification of pediatric injuries is shown in Figure 8.16.

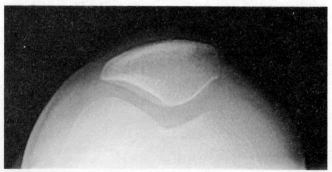

Figure 8.15 Sunrise (Merchant) view of the knee.

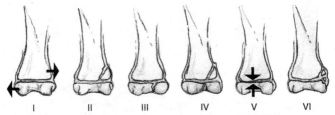

Figure 8.16 Salter-Harris classification of epiphyseal fractures.

Tibial Plateau Fractures

These fractures are very common in the setting of axial-loading injuries. Motor-vehicle accidents, long falls onto the feet, and automobile versus pedestrian accidents are frequent causes. The Schatzker classification reflects the fact that most fractures of this type involve the lateral tibial condyle. Medial condylar involvement implies a more significant mechanism of injury. The surrounding structures that are susceptible to injury include the medial and lateral menisci, the cruciate ligament, and posterior displacement, which endangers the popliteal artery. Plain-film radiographs in three views (AP, lateral, and oblique) usually are sufficient; however, CT often is necessary to correctly image the fracture and to plan operative management.

Unhappy Triad

This term describes a collection of injuries that are common to athletes such as skiers and football players. Traumatic force applied to the lateral aspect of the knee results in a torn ACL, medial meniscus, and MCL. The most disabling of these injuries is the torn ACL, which is a primary stabilizer of anterior and posterior forces—specifically, forward translation of the tibia at the knee joint. Women are more susceptible than men to ACL injury but may be less likely to engage in vigorous contact sports. This is a classic however incorrect depiction of this combination of knee injuries. The lateral meniscus is more often injured in complex knee injuries.

SELECTED DISORDERS OF THE KNEE

Compartment Syndrome

In compartment syndrome (Fig. 8.17), fascial compartment pressures exceed the blood pressure, keeping the perfusing capillaries open. If this persists, the risk of permanent ischemic contractures increases. The "worst-case" scenario is one that involves enough muscle and tissue necrosis to provoke rhabdomyolysis and acute tubular necrosis. The limbs and fascial compartments are most affected, followed by

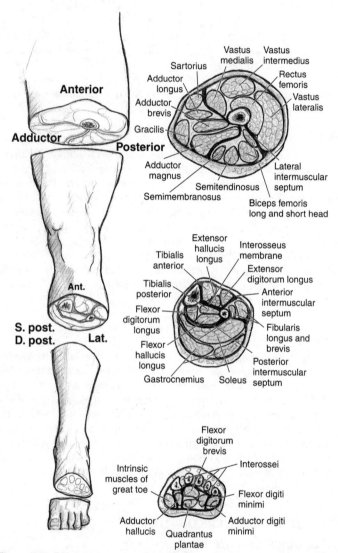

Figure 8.17 Fascial compartment of the thigh, lower leg, and foreleg.

the forearm and, uncommonly, the foot and thigh. Compartment syndrome often is characterized by the **5 P's: P**ain (with passive extension), **P**allor, **P**ressure, **P**aresthesia, and **P**ulselessness. It often follows severe lower-leg crush injuries of the tibia. Pressures are checked via a large needle with a pressure apparatus (Stryker needle), and values greater than 30–40 should raise the suspicion of compartment syndrome and indicate the need for fasciotomy.

Anserine Bursitis

The knee has 12 bursae, one of which underlies the attachment of the pes anserinus as it runs over the MCL. The bursa is located approximately 3 cm below the tibial plateau. Pain and inflammation of the bursa are common, especially in the presence of osteoarthritis. Treatment for this condition is the same as that for all bursitis: rest, nonsteroidal anti-inflammatory drugs (NSAIDs), corticosteroid injections, and physiotherapy.

Patellofemoral Joint Disorders

Patellar pain can result from many causes, such as trauma and repetitive-use trauma, or have no perceptible etiology. Dislocation and subluxation often are apparent to the patient and can be elicited in the history, but disorders of patellar tracking in the femoral condylar groove may not be obvious. Previous fractures can lead to malalignment or spur formation. Tendonitis can be present in knee-dependent athletes and weight lifters. Evaluation should focus on normal movement, crepitus, and muscular development surrounding the knee, especially the vastus medialis oblique fibers (or VMO insufficiency). Plain-film radiographs and MRI aid in establishing the diagnosis but cannot replace a good physical examination. Treatment is aimed largely at physiotherapy and strengthening exercises, including electromyelography, to build knee support. Braces can be helpful in the short term. Surgical options include arthroscopic débridement and patellar replacement or resurfacing.

Primary Tumors of Bone

Although these tumors are very uncommon—an average orthopaedist can expect to encounter one case every 5 years—they are nonetheless an important topic. Metastatic disease is the much more common tumor of bone and needs to be differentiated from primary tumors, especially in women, because breast cancer is the most common primary site. The patient with a bone lesion most likely is

Table 8.6 Cartilage- and Bone-Forming Tumors

Cartilaginous Tumors	Osteoid-Forming Tumors
Osteochondroma	Osteoma
Enchondroma	Osteoid osteoma
Chondroblastoma	Osteoblastoma
Chondrosarcoma	Osteosarcoma

young and presents with pain, swelling, tenderness, and fractures related to minor trauma. Although all of these tumors are of mesenchymal origin, they can be divided into cartilage-forming and bone-forming lesions and further classified as benign or malignant (Tables 8.6 and 8.7).

Proceeding in order from the most common to the least common are multiple myeloma, osteosarcoma, chondrosarcoma, and Ewing's sarcoma, which are all malignant tumors. Osteochondromas and giant cell tumors of bone are the most frequently encountered benign tumors. The age of presentation and rate of onset of symptoms are helpful factors in guiding the differential from primary to metastatic and from benign to malignant. The presence of a cortical bone capsule implies a benign process that has been chronic, whereas the inability to distinguish areas of pathogenic bone growth from normal bone implies malignancy.

Table 8.7 Characteristics of Benign and Malignant Primary Bone Tumors

Benign	Malignant
Cystic mass with rim of mature cortex	Bone destruction with loss of continuity. No good distinguishing characteristics between normal and abnormal bone
Definable cortical capsule, cancellous or cortical bone loss within	Large areas of bone loss without encapsulation
No new periosteal bone reformation	Multiple layers of bone or periosteal formation (onion-skinning) or spiculated (sunburst) linear calcifications

Tests that should be part of the differential diagnosis include:

Alkaline phosphatase: Elevated in 50% of osteosarcomas.

Prostate-specific antigen and acid phosphatase: Can rule out prostate cancer.

Lactate dehydrogenase and erythrocyte sedimentation rate: Often elevated in Ewing's sarcoma.

Calcium and phosphate. Affected in all cases of bone formation or destruction.

Thyroid function tests: Can rule out thyroid cancer.

Serum and urine protein electrophoresis: Can be used to differentiate from myeloma.

Complete blood count: An increased white blood cell count can indicate osteomyelitis.

Bone scan: May be helpful to identify other lesions.

CT and MRI: Can be helpful in establishing the diagnosis and extent of destruction as well as associated soft tissue masses.

Chest radiography or CT: Used to look for possible metastasis.

Chemotherapy with radiation and adequate excision or amputation of the affected limb are the general means for treatment of malignant tumors. These techniques usually are not indicated in benign tumors, because radiation can increase the risk of other tumors, such as osteogenic sarcoma.

Benign Tumors

Osteoid osteoma: Like most bone tumors, this is found primarily in the young. It characteristically manifests as a dull, aching pain at night that is relieved by aspirin, which acts on prostaglandins within the tumor nidus. This has led to some controversy regarding whether this is an inflammatory process (e.g., Brodie's abscess) or a true neoplasm. These tumors are small (up to 1 cm) and inspire reactive bone formation around the tumor foci, forming a dense, sclerotic bone capsule. Common sites are the femur and spine. Treatment is primarily via NSAIDs or aspirin but can include surgical resection if refractory to drugs.

Osteochondroma: The most common benign primary tumor of bone, this most often is found in the metaphysis of long bones (distal femur and humerus) in children and in young adults up to 20 years of age. Lesions consist of lobulated, bony stalks with cartilaginous caps that grow in childhood and then stop. An autosomal dominant version of this tumor also exists and presents as multiple osteochondromas (also called bony exostoses); it is associated with an increased incidence of progression to chondrosarcoma.

Enchondromas: These benign cartilaginous tumors most often occur in the intramedullary areas of tubular bones of the hands. Again, there is an increased risk of sarcomatous progression with multiple tumors, as in disorders such as Ollier's disease and Maffucci's syndrome.

Giant cell tumors of bone: In contrast to the other bone tumors, giant cell tumors occur primarily in adults and predominantly in women. Finding an aneurysmal bone cyst should raise the suspicion of a giant cell tumor, because the two often occur together. The radiographic findings show characteristic "soap bubble" areas of bone destruction that begin in the epiphysis and extend toward the diaphysis. The neoplastic component of the tumor is a mesenchymal stromal cell and not the multinucleated giant cell; therefore, little bone formation occurs around the soft tumor mass without calcification. These tumors have a tendency to recur. Surgical removal is the treatment of choice except in the spine and sacrum, where radiation may have a place.

Malignant Tumors

Osteogenic sarcoma: This is not only the most common malignant bone tumor but also perhaps the most aggressive. Occurring mostly in children and young adults, with a male predominance (3:2), osteosarcomas usually are found in the metaphysis of long bones near the knee and elbow joints. The metaphysis of the distal femur is the most common location. Much has been said of the characteristic "sunburst" spiculated, "hair-on-end" radiograph, including elevation of the periosteum producing a "Codman's triangle," although these are not specific to osteosarcomas. Chemotherapy plus resection and amputation are the treatments of choice. Radiation/chemotherapy without amputation currently is being researched and may be indicated in the future. Osteosarcomas are associated with radiation treatment secondary to other disorders, such as Paget's disease of bone, retinoblastoma, and avascular necrosis of infracted bone. Osteosarcoma is another neoplasm that can express the Her-2/neu (human epidermal growth factor receptor), which indicates a more aggressive form of the disease. However, this also may increase susceptibility to the drug trastuzumab (Herceptin) via antibody-dependent cytotoxicity. Chest radiographs should be included in the evaluation to rule out metastatic disease.

Chondrosarcoma: This tumor may mimic the characteristics of osteosarcoma in its presentation and radiologic findings. Chondrosarcomas have a male predominance (2:1) and are approximately half as frequent as osteosarcomas. The sites most favored by the tumor are the pelvis, ribs, and scapula. In contrast to osteosarcoma, radiation and chemotherapy have only limited or questionable therapeutic efficacy, and complete surgical resection is necessary to prevent recurrence.

Ewing's sarcoma: This is another pediatric, male-predominant tumor (3:2) that most often affects the lower extremities and pelvis. Known to medical students as one of the small blue cell tumors (others include acute leukemia, mesothelioma, neuroblastoma, rhabdomyosarcoma, and Wilms' tumor), it also is notable for it association with a t(11;22) translocation. This tumor may present in children as a infection-like process with fever, inflammation at the tumor site, and anemia.

Quick Look • Knee

Inspect the skin, looking for gross deformity, effusion, guarding, or bruising.

Palpate and attempt to locate the area of greatest pain; medializing or lateralizing pain, above or below the patella; help narrow the differential diagnosis before imaging.

Attempt to move the knee through its range of motion. In the "status post–knee replacement" patient, this can be a measure of success.

- **Flexion:** 135°.
- **Extension:** 0–5°.
- **Internal rotation:** 10°.
- **External rotation:** 10°.

Reflex testing if neurologic deficits, cervical stenosis, or upper motor neuron (UMN)/lower motor neuron (LMN) disorder is suspected or if the patient is preoperative or postoperative.

- **Patellar (L4), Achilles (S1).**
  - **Absent:** Neuropathy, LMN lesion.
  - **Hyperactive:** UMN lesion.

Evaluate muscles using **special tests** to isolate the disorder.

- **Apley test:** Medial and lateral meniscal tears. Patient lies prone with the knee flexed. Press down on the heel, and rotate the tibia.
- **Anterior drawer test:** ACL insufficiency. Pull the tibia forward and away from femur in a 90° flexed knee.
- **Apprehension test:** Patellar dislocation and subluxation. Try to laterally dislocate the patella.
- **Ballottement test:** Knee effusion. Push the patella into the trochlear groove.
- **Bounce home test:** Swelling in a joint. Flex the knee in an elevated leg. The leg should fall straight.
- **Bulge sign:** Minor knee effusion. Press the lateral aspect of the knee, and observe for a medial knee bulge.
- **Distraction test:** Distinguishes between meniscal and ligamentous damage. Pull upward in traction and rotate tibia. Pain suggests a ligament tear.
- **External rotation recurvatum test:** PCL insufficiency. Pick up the extended leg by the foot.
- **Lachman test:** ACL insufficiency. Pull the tibia forward and away from femur in a 30° flexed knee.
- **McMurray test:** Posterior meniscal tears. Apply valgus stress while externally rotating the bent knee in a supine patient.
- **Posterior drawer test:** PCL insufficiency. Push the tibia backward and away from the femur in a 90° flexed knee.
- **Quadriceps active test:** PCL tear. Fire the quadriceps in an approximately 80° flexed knee. Apply posterior stress on the tibia at the ankle joint.
- **Pivot shift test:** ACL insufficiency. Place valgus stress at the knee joint, with some internal rotation, while moving knee though flexion at the knee joint.
- **Varus/valgus test:** In a 30° flexed knee, apply varus and valgus to assess collateral laxity.
  - **Positive varus laxity:** LCL weakness/tear.
  - **Positive valgus laxity:** MCL weakness/tear

Order appropriate radiographs.

- **AP:** Are the intercondylar eminences centered between the femoral condyles? The femoral condyles are not rotated, with equal medial and lateral joint spaces; patella is midline.
  - Follow the tibial cortex, and scrutinize the trabeculae and supracondylar femur for fracture, impaction, or unexplained densities.
  - Examine the margin of the patella under hot light.

- **Lateral:** Note rotated, and the femoral condyles will be in line with nearly complete overlap. The fibula is separate, and the AP margins of the tibia and fibula are distinct.
  - Visualize the AP surface of the condyles.
  - Evaluate the patella using the Insall-Salvati ratio if necessary.
- **Sunrise (Merchant) view:** Vertical patellar fractures are visible. Is the patella sitting in the groove?
- **Oblique views:** Fractures of the femoral condyles and tibial plateau?

SELECTED REFERENCES

Felder CR, Leeson MA. Patellofemoral Pain Syndrome: The Use of Electromyographic Biofeedback for Training the Vastus Medialis Obliquus in Patients with Patellofemoral Pain. Available at: http://www.bfe.org/protocol/pro01eng.htm. Accessed November 21, 2005.

Marx JA. Rosen's Emergency Medicine: Concepts and Clinical Practice, 5th ed. St. Louis: Mosby; 2002.

Randall RL. Tumors in orthopaedics. In: Current Diagnosis and Treatment in Orthopaedics, 3rd Ed. New York: McGraw Hill (Lange), 2003:286–348.

Reveille JD. Soft-tissue rheumatism: diagnosis and treatment. Am J Med 1997;102:23S–29S.

Simon MA, Finn HA. Diagnostic strategy for bone and soft-tissue tumors. J Bone Joint Surg Am 1993;75:622–632.

9

Foot and Ankle

ANATOMY

Bony and Ligamentous Anatomy

The anatomy of the foot is shown in Figure 9.1. Specific bones and joints of the foot and ankle include:

Talus: This key bone transfers weight from the body to the calcaneus. It has no muscular or tendinous attachments of its own. Tendons destined for the calcaneus pass through the sulcus tali. This is the most commonly injured joint in the body, most often at the anterior talofibular and calcaneofibular ligament via an inversion injury. Eversion injuries are much less common but can result in disruption of the medial (deltoid) ligament and transferred force, fracturing the fibula (Pott's fracture). In an ankle sprain, the lateral aspect is the site of inversion plantar injury (Table 9.1). In pes planus ("flat foot"), the talar head displaces medially and plantarward.

Talocrural joint: The talar dome forms a ginglymus (hinge) articulation with the distal tibia and fibula and is the principal joint of the ankle. It contains an articular capsule anteriorly and posteriorly. This ankle mortise joint is wider anteriorly and is convex from front to back and concave from side to side. The tibiotalar ligament also is called the deltoid ligament and is the key structure preventing excessive eversion.

Talocalcaneal joint: This subtalar synovial joint has its own articular capsule that is predominantly responsible for eversion and inversion. Fractures of the talocrural and subtalar joints are serious injuries and imply considerable axial loading.

Talocalcaneonavicular joint: This joint plays an important role in preserving the arch of the foot. Together with the calcaneocuboid joint, it forms the transverse tarsal joint, which is responsible for eversion and inversion of the foot.

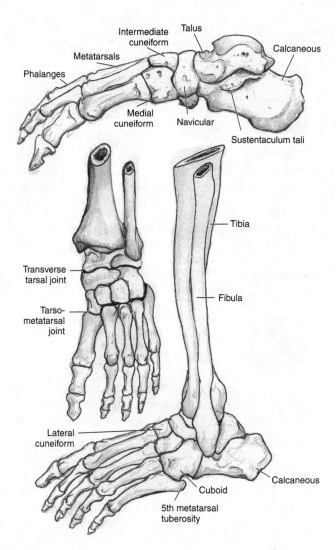

Figure 9.1 Anterior foot.

Table 9.1 Ligaments of the Lateral Malleolus

Anterior
Anterior talofibular ligament
Calcaneofibular ligament
Posterior
Posterior talofibular ligament

Calcaneus: This is the largest, strongest bone in the foot. As with the talus, fracture implies considerable axial loading. The sustentaculum tali is the medial arch that supports part of the talus and transmits the flexor hallucis longus tendon.

Navicular: The navicular articulates posteriorly with the talus (talonavicular), anteriorly with the three cuneiforms, and laterally with the cuboid.

Cuboid: This is part of the transverse tarsal joint and the keystone in the lateral longitudinal arch of the foot via the plantar calcaneocuboid ligament.

Cuneiforms: The medial three tarsal bones articulate with the navicular bone posteriorly and the first three metatarsal bones anteriorly.

Metatarsals: The base of the fifth metatarsal forms the most palpable prominence of the metatarsal bones and is a frequent site of avulsion fractures. The head of the fifth metatarsal is the site of lateral bursitis (tailor's bunion). The first metatarsal has both a medial and a lateral sesamoid bone just inferior to the head. The first metatarsal joint is the most frequent site of gouty arthritis, also called podagra. The second metatarsal joint has little movement, and subjecting it to uncommon use can result in fatigue "march" fractures. The head of the first metatarsal is the site of hallux valgus metatarsus primus varus, which is a medial angulation of the first metatarsal shaft. It can cause a bursa to form, which irritates and leads to formation of a bunion (differential diagnosis is gouty tophi).

Phalanges: As in the hands, the great toe has only two bones. Flexion of the metatarsophalangeal (MTP) joint and extension of the interphalangeal joint is present in a "hammer toe."

Tendons and Soft Tissue

The medial malleolus tendons from anterior to posterior (Fig. 9.2) are:

Tom	**T**ibialis Posterior
Dick	Flexor **D**igitorum Longus
And	Posterior Tibial **A**rtery and Tibial **n**erve
Harry	Flexor **H**allucis Longus

Note: Medial malleolar tendons have a synovial sheath, which can become inflamed. This is known as synovitis.

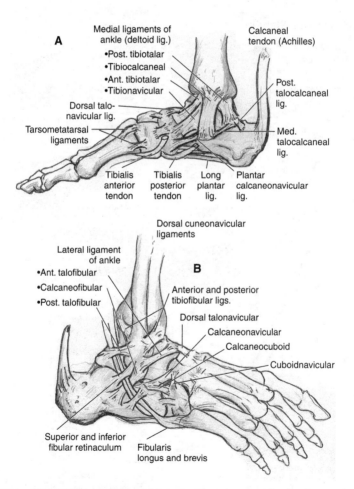

Figure 9.2 Medial (**a**) and lateral (**b**) views of foot. Ant., anterior; lig., ligament; med., medial; Post., posterior.

Dorsum of the Foot

Medially, the dorsum of the foot includes the tibialis anterior tendon, extensor hallucis longus (EHL) tendon, and the dorsal pedal artery. Laterally, it includes the extensor digitorum longus (EDL) tendon.

The EHL can be transferred to the plantar aspect of the foot to correct a footdrop. The EHL tendons also mark the site of anterior compartment syndrome ("March syndrome"). The dorsalis pedis artery is between the EHL and the EDL.

Ankle Joint Stability

Injury (Fig. 9.3) caused by excessive inversion is more common for two reasons:

1. The medial malleolus is shorter, which predisposes the talus to inversion more than to eversion.
2. Lateral ligaments are thicker but not as strong as the large deltoid medial ligament.

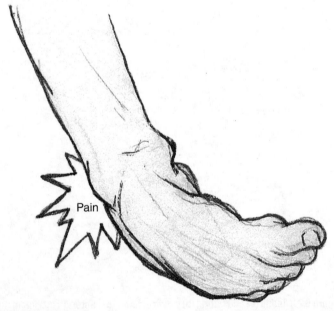

Pain

Figure 9.3 Ankle sprain.

Note: The talus can now slide forward on the tibia (the anterior talofibular ligament prevents subluxation of the talus).

Muscular Anatomy

Table 9.2 outlines the basic muscular organization and innervation of the ankle and foot. Figure 9.4 shows how the muscles are arranged in the ankle and foot. Table 9.3 names the primary dorsiflexors and the primary plantar flexors of the ankle and foot.

Vascular and Neuroanatomy

The tibial nerve travels in a tarsal tunnel, which can be impinged in a carpal tunnel–like process. The saphenous vein is immediately anterior to the medial malleolus.

BASIC EXAMINATION

The field of podiatry takes comfort in the difficult examination of the foot (job security), which, much like the hand, is a high-yield site of injury and pathology. Neurovascular status should always be checked to rule out vascular insufficiency by palpating the distal and posterior tibial pulses. The foot should be taken through its range of motion (ROM) by dorsiflexing and plantar flexing the ankle and toe joints as well as everting and inverting the ankle. Midfoot abduction and adduction can be used to assess the calcaneocuboid and talonavicular joints. Always compare ROM bilaterally. Table 9.4 may be used to help limit the differential diagnosis.

Extensor (dorsiflexor) tendons cross the ankle and are easily injured; they travel behind the lateral malleolus and can subluxate or tear. Evertors often are injured in the familiar "ankle sprain" (Fig. 9.3). In contrast, invertors and the plantar flexors travel behind the medial malleolus. Pain often is present one finger below the lateral malleolus. The posterior tibial tendon also is prone to tenosynovitis and can rupture. Palpation of the plantar fascia while dorsiflexing the toes can rule out plantar fasciitis. The MTP joint is the primary site for onset of gout. The sustentaculum tali is one finger below the medial malleolus and is the attachment for the spring ligament. The peroneus brevis inserts at the base of the fifth metatarsal and usually should prompt radiography of the foot in ankle sprains to rule out a common avulsion fracture of the fifth metatarsal. The sinus tarsi is the soft depression just anterior to the lateral malleolus, the site of a subtalar arthrodesis. The medial tubercle of the calcaneus is the site of a heel spur.

(text continues on p. 242)

Table 9.2 Muscles of the Ankle and Foot[a]

Muscle	Nerve (Root)	Origin	Insertion
Ankle			
Anterior compartment			
Tibialis anterior	Deep fibular (L4 and L5)	Lateral condyle, lateral tibia	First metatarsal, medial cuneiform
Extensor hallucis longus	Deep fibular (L5 and S1)	Anterior fibula	Base of great toe
Extensor digitorum longus	Deep fibular (L5 and S1)	Lateral tibial condyle, anterior fibula	Bases of phalanges 2–5
Fibularis tertius	Deep fibular (L5 and S1)	Inferior anterior fibula	Dorsal base of fifth metatarsal
Lateral compartment			
Fibularis longus	Superficial peroneal (L5 and S1)	Fibular head, superior half	Base of first metatarsal, medial cuneiform
Fibularis brevis	Superficial peroneal (L5 and S1)	Inferior half of fibula	Base of fifth metatarsal, lateral aspect
Superficial posterior compartment			
Gastrocnemius	Tibial (S1 and S2)	Lateral head: Lateral femoral condyle Medial head: Posterior supracondylar (popliteal) fossa	Posterior calcaneus (via Achilles tendon)

(continued on next page)

Muscle	Innervation	Proximal Attachment	Distal Attachment
Soleus	Tibial (S1 and S2)	Fibular head, posterior fibula, medial tibia	Posterior calcaneus (via Achilles tendon)
Plantaris	Tibial (S1 and S2)	Lateral supracondylar ridge	Posterior calcaneus (via Achilles tendon)
Deep posterior compartment			
Popliteus	Tibial (L4 and L5)	Lateral femoral condyle	Posterior superior tibia
Flexor hallucis longus	Tibial (S2 and S3)	Posterior inferior fibula	Base of distal great toe
Flexor digitorum longus	Tibial (S2 and S3)	Posterior fibula	Bases of distal phalanges 2–5
Tibialis posterior	Tibial (L4 and L5)	Interosseous membrane, posterior tibia and fibula	Plantar navicular, cuboid, cuneiform, metatarsals 2–4
Foot			
Dorsum			
Extensor digitorum brevis	Deep fibular nerve	Dorsal calcaneus	Extensor digitorum longus tendon
Extensor hallucis brevis	Deep fibular nerve	Dorsal calcaneus	Base of great toe
Sole			
[1]Adductor hallucis	Medial plantar nerve (S2 and S3)	Medial calcaneal tubercle	Medial base of great toe
[1]Flexor digitorum brevis	Medial plantar nerve (S2 and S3)	Medial calcaneal tubercle	Phalanges 2–5
[1]Adductor digiti minimi	Lateral plantar nerve (S2 and S3)	Medial and lateral calcaneal tubercle	Lateral base of fifth phalanx

(continued on next page)

Table 9.2 Muscles of the Ankle and Foot[a] (*Continued*)

Muscle	Nerve (Root)	Origin	Insertion
[2]Quadratus plantae	Lateral plantar nerve (S2 and S3)	Medial and lateral calcaneus	Flexor digitorum longus tendon
[2]Lumbricals	Medial and lateral plantar nerve (S2 and S3)	Flexor digitorum longus tendon	Medial bases of phalanges 2–5, flexor digitorum longus expansion
[3]Flexor hallucis brevis	Medial plantar nerve (S2/S3)	Cuboid, lateral cuneiforms	Base of great toe (both sides)
[3]Adductor hallucis	Deep lateral plantar nerve (S2 and S3)	Base of metatarsals 2–4, metatarsophalangeal ligaments	Lateral base of great toe
[3]Flexor digiti minimi	Superficial lateral plantar nerve (S2 and S3)	Base of fifth metatarsal	Base of fifth phalanx
[4]Plantar interossei	Lateral plantar nerve (S2 and S3)	Base of metatarsals 3–5	Base of proximal phalanges 3–5
[4]Dorsal interossei	Lateral plantar nerve (S2 and S3)	Sides of metatarsals 1–5	Proximal phalanx, second digit; lateral aspect of phalanges 2–4

[a]Superscript numbers [1,2,3,4] refer to the relative level/depth of the muscles of the plantar foot.

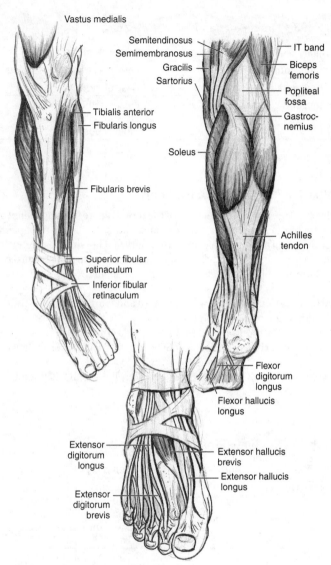

Figure 9.4 Vascular and neuroanatomic illustrations of the lower leg.

Table 9.3 Dorsiflexors and Plantar Flexors

Primary Dorsiflexors	Primary Plantar Flexors
Tibialis anterior	Peroneus longus and brevis
Extensor hallucis longus	Gastrocnemius and soleus
Extensor digitorum longus	Flexor hallucis longus Flexor digitorum longus Tibialis posterior

Palpation (Soft Tissue of the Foot)

Palpate all the bony prominences of the foot. Palpate the calcaneus for bursitis of the retrocalcaneal or calcaneal bursa. The fifth metatarsal base and head are high-yield areas for injury and bursitis, respectively. Palpate all joints for warmth or pain, and palpate the plantar surface.

Points to bear in mind during palpation include:

- **Morton's neuroma:** Between the third and fourth metatarsal heads.
- **Point tenderness:** Plantar fasciitis.
- **Discrete palpable nodules:** Dupuytren's contracture.
- **Claw toes:** Hyperextension of MTP and the distal interphalangeal (DIP).
- **Hammer toes:** Flexion of proximal interphalangeal (PIP) joint.

Table 9.4 Differential Diagnosis of Foot Pathology

Disorder	Age	Sex	Deformity
Osteoarthritis	50–80	Female	Flexion and lateral deviation of proximal interphalangeal (PIP) and distal interphalangeal, Heberden's nodes
Rheumatoid arthritis	5–80+	Female	Flexion of metacarpophalangeal and PIP, ulnar deviation (swan neck, boutonnière)
Gout	25–85	Male	Uncommon, tophi (usually in feet)
Reiter's syndrome	10–80	Male	Swelling of ankle, heel, and toes

Range of Motion

To test active ROM of the foot and ankle:

- **Plantar flexion and toe motion:** Walk on toes.
- **Dorsiflexion:** Walk on heels.
- **Inversion:** Walk on lateral borders.
- **Eversion:** Walk on medial borders.

For flexion:

Ankle mortise	50°
First MTP	40°

For extension:

Ankle mortise	15°
First MTP	60–75°
Inversion (subtalar)	20°
Eversion (subtalar)	10°

Points to bear in mind during ROM testing include:

- Decreased intermalleolar distance limits dorsiflexion (i.e., swelling, fusion, contracture, or interarticular swelling caused by trauma or edema).
- Inversion and eversion test of the talocalcaneal, talonavicular, talocuboid.
- Adduction and abduction test of the talonavicular and talocuboid
- First MTP joint with reduced ROM indicates hallux rigidus.

Perform the following tests:

Tibialis Anterior: Heel walk with inversion, or hang ankles while dorsiflexing and everting.

Extensor Hallucis Longus: Heel walk and resist dorsiflexion at the DIP joint (the PIP joint is EHB).

Ext. Digitorum Longus: Fanning toes up against resistance.

Ext. Hallucis Brevis: Cannot be isolated; same as EHL.

Peroneus Longus & Peroneus Brevis: Walk on medial the borders of the feet, or resist plantar flexion and eversion.

G & S: Calf raises.

Flexor Hallucis Longus: Observe toe-off gait, or oppose great toe plantar flexion.

Flexor Digitorum Longus: Great toe flexion.

Tibialis Posterior: Difficult to isolate; resist plantar flexion and eversion.

Sensation

Figure 9.5 is a vascular and neuroanatomic illustration of the lower leg. Figure 9.6 illustrates the Achilles reflex.

Note: An alternate method for testing Achilles reflex if pain or swelling is present is to press against the ball of the foot to dorsiflex and strike the fingers with a hammer.

SPECIAL TESTS

Ankle Dorsiflexion Test

The ankle dorsiflexion test determines whether the gastrocnemius or the gastrocnemius–soleus is limiting motion:

1. Flex the knee joint. If you cannot dorsiflex the ankle, then the gastrocnemius is limiting (flexion slackens the gastrocnemius, a two-joint spanning muscle).
2. The soleus should be the same in either flexion or extension (a one-joint muscle).

Anterior Drawer Test

The anterior drawer test (Fig. 9.7) is a test of ankle instability. Flex the patient's knee, stabilize the tibia by cupping the heel, and move the ankle mortise joint in an anteroposterior direction. A positive test is asymmetric ankle excursion.

Flat Feet Test

Observe the arch while the patient is sitting and standing.

Forefoot Adduction Test

Forefoot adduction (Fig. 9.8) is common condition in children. A correction test determines if the angle needs to be corrected. If the foot cannot be abducted beyond a neutral position, then correction is advised.

Homan's Test

Pain in the calf (especially following surgery) with forced dorsiflexion in addition to pain on palpation suggests, with low specificity, a possible deep venous thrombosis (DVT). Actually, in Homan's original

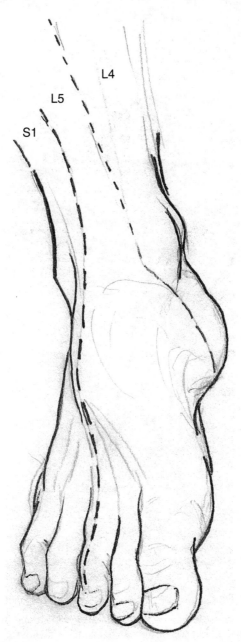

Figure 9.5 Foot dermatome.

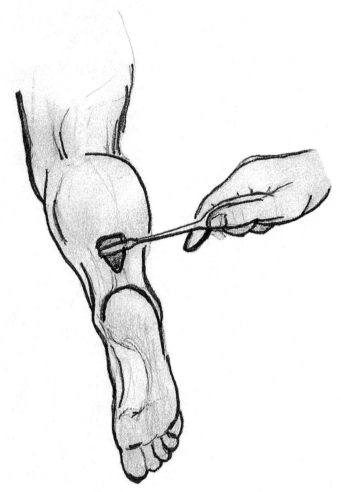

Figure 9.6 Achilles reflex.

paper, the positive test was a spinal reflex to rapid dorsiflexion in trans-Atlantic pilots with deep venous thrombosus (DVT).

Talar Tilt Test

The talar tilt test indicates ankle instability. Inversion at the ankle causes tilting and lifting of the mortise joint. A positive test is asymmetric ankle excursion.

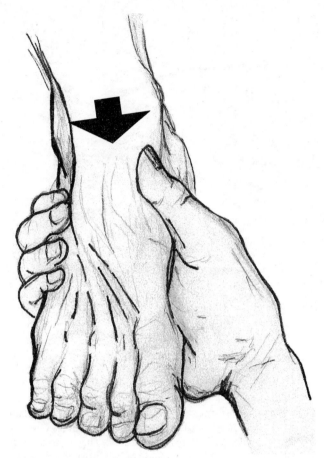

Figure 9.7 Anterior drawer test.

Thompson Test

The Thompson test (Fig. 9.9) is a test for Achilles tendon rupture/tear. Flex the knee in a prone patient; squeezing the calf should provoke plantar flexion. A positive test is no plantar flexion.

Tibial Torsion (Toeing-In)

An imaginary line drawn between the malleoli is rotated 15° from a perpendicular line drawn from the tibial tubercle to the ankle. The ankle mortise in internal tibial torsion faces anteriorly or internally.

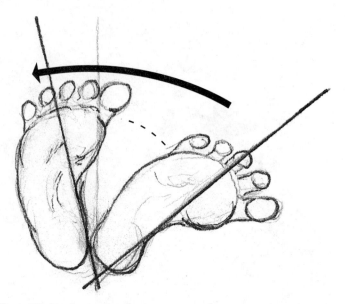

Figure 9.8 Forefront adduction test.

RADIOLOGIC APPROACH TO THE FOOT AND ANKLE
Overview

The foot and ankle are commonly imaged structures, and many unnecessary studies are performed in the name of ankle and foot pain. As with the knee, many attempts have been made to minimize radiography in the foot and ankle (e.g., Ottawa ankle rules). These and other treatment algorithms have studied foot and ankle injury patterns and identified common indicators of fractures versus soft tissue injuries.

The Ottawa ankle rules identify four areas of point tenderness:

- The most distal 6 cm of the posterior (not anterior) aspects of the medial and lateral malleolus.
- The base of the fifth metatarsal.
- The navicular bone.

Also included is the inability to bear weight since the injury. This symptom is not valid, however, in cases with distracting injuries, altered mentation, or intoxication.

Areas of high suspicion should be examined carefully in the radiographic series of the foot and ankle. Both malleoli should be viewed

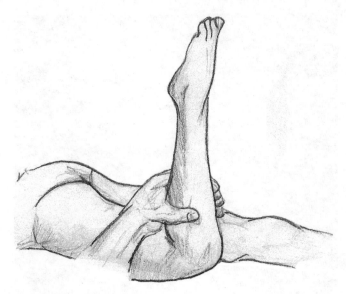

Figure 9.9 Thompson test.

closely, including the posterior aspect of the tibia (posterior malleoli), and using a hot light if necessary.

Views

Note: Check to make sure you have the correct patient, the correct date, and the correct anatomy.

Ankle

Lateral View

Although there is considerable overlap of the ankle bones, the lateral view (Fig. 9.10) provides a clear view of the anteroposterior (AP) margins of the tibia and fibula. Specifically:

* Pay close attention to the fifth metatarsal base for an avulsion fracture.
* The talar dome should appear as a smooth arc; disruption indicates a tibial plafond fracture.

Anteroposterior View

The AP view (Fig. 9.11) is standard and provides good visualization of the distal tibia and fibula. The ankle mortise joint is visible, although it is

(text continues on p. 252)

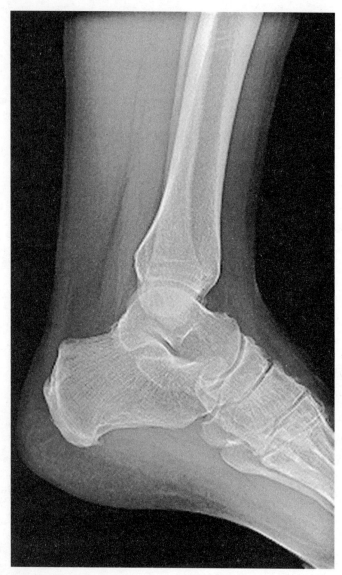

Figure 9.10 Lateral radiograph of the ankle.

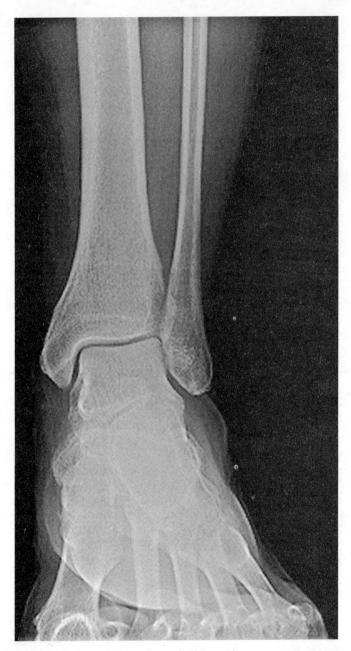

Figure 9.11 Anteroposterior radiograph of the ankle.

obscured by bony overlap. For a complete view without any overlap of the ankle joint, a mortise view can be shot with 15° of internal rotation.

When examining an AP view:

- Identify the clear area between the talar dome and lateral malleolus, indicating no rotation.
- Follow the cortices of the tibia and fibula as well as the tibial plafond (articulation with the talar dome).

Mortise View

The mortise view (Fig. 9.12) is the definitive view of the ankle mortise joint. Examine this view with a hot light if necessary to inspect for bone fragments. Specifically:

- Any widening of the joint space may indicate a fractured malleolus or disruption of the ankle ligaments. The normal joint space should be uniform in width.
- The medial clear space should be intact and not wide (<4 mm).
- Inspect the dome of the talus.
- The lateral tibiofibular clear space should be less than 5.5 mm.

Foot

As with the ankle, examination findings in the foot such as point tenderness and inability to bear weight are more sensitive findings than soft tissue swelling or bruising. The mechanism of injury is always important. For instance, a fall from a height onto the feet can anticipate calcaneal fractures or other axial loading injuries. As always, scrutinize areas of concern based on the physical examination findings.

Three views are standard: the AP, the lateral, and the internal oblique. The internal oblique is added to see all the MTP articulations not depicted on the AP view. An additional coned-down view of the calcaneus, talus, midfoot, and toes can be obtained if these are not well depicted on standard views. Approach each view of the foot in the same systematic manner as the others (e.g., hindfoot, midfoot, or forefoot) so that the same structures are always identified.

Anteroposterior View

The only unobscured view of the first and second MTP joints is the AP. When examining an AP view:

- Check the alignment of the navicular bone with the talus. The midtarsal joints (calcaneocuboid and talonavicular) should be checked for fracture.

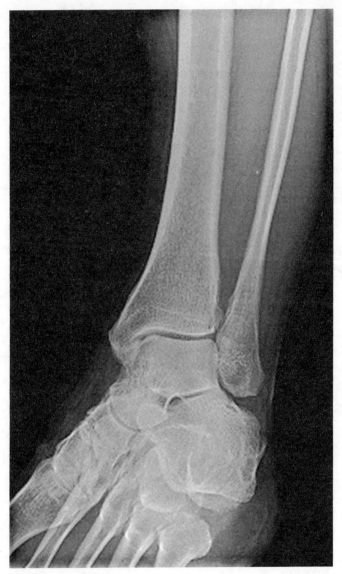

Figure 9.12 Oblique radiograph of the ankle.

- The lateral cortex of the second metatarsal should align with the lateral aspect of the second cuneiform. The lateral is useful for determining translation in a dislocation. The first through third metatarsal bases can be viewed.
- Scan the phalanges and metatarsals.
- All other bone cortices should be smooth and intact.

Lateral View

The lateral view of the foot is important. Start back to front (or front to back) and be mindful of the common areas of concern: the talus, calcaneus, talar body and neck, metatarsal alignment, and fifth metatarsal base.

When examining a lateral view:

- Inspect the talar dome and subtalar joint. The talar neck is a common site of fracture in motor-vehicle accidents.
- Evaluate the calcaneus for fracture. Calculate the Bohler's angle, which will be less than 20° in most depressed calcaneal fractures. Fractures to look for include those of the anterior process, body, and tuberosity.
- The os trigonum is an unfused accessory ossicle and normal variant.
- Examine the base of the fifth metatarsal for an avulsion or occult fracture.

Internal Oblique View

This slightly angled projection shows the metatarsal bases that are not well depicted in the AP view. Again, scan the film from back to front (or front to back), identifying all of the bones of the foot as you go. Specifically:

- The anterior talar neck is seen well.
- Additional angles of the calcaneus can be seen. Scan the anterior process for fracture or avulsion fragments.
- Check the intertarsal and tarsometatarsal joints for symmetry and congruence.
- Check the metatarsals and phalanges for fracture. Jones and pseudo-Jones fractures of the fifth metatarsal base and tuberosity are best seen in this view.
- The medial border of the fourth metatarsal should align with the medial cortex of the cuboid.

SELECTED FRACTURES OF THE FOOT AND ANKLE

Calcaneal Fracture

The calcaneal fracture is the most frequent fracture of the foot. Fractures of the calcaneus are often comminuted and imply significant axial loading or twisting forces. Injuries further downstream in the transmission of force should be assessed for knee and spinal injuries. Because of the heavy demands that are put on the foot, these fractures heal poorly, and surgical management is difficult. The radiographic evaluation should include calculation of Bohler's and Gissane's angles on the lateral view. A Bohler's angle of less than 25–30° can indicate a posterior facet fracture. A Gissane's angle of greater than 125–140° also is associated with the collapse of the posterior facet. The initial management should include immobilization of the ankle in a Robert Jones (bulky Jones) dressing. This dressing is composed of several layers of soft cast padding (Webril) and a thick cotton roll, secured by a posterior slab (fiberglass or plaster), and surrounded by a woven elastic (Ace) bandage. Classification of these fractures first focuses on whether they involve the talocalcaneal joint. Further classification follows well-established fracture patterns according to several schemes. Surgical management often is necessary and seeks to reestablish the subtalar joint, Bohler's angle, and width of the calcaneus. These patients often are plagued by issues of chronic pain despite good surgical approximation.

Fifth Metatarsal Fracture (Jones and Pseudo-Jones)

This avulsion of the peroneus brevis tendon (pseudo-Jones) from its attachment to the base of the fifth metatarsal bone usually results from a sudden inversion injury and is a common fracture. These should be distinguished from Jones fractures (Fig. 9.13), which are fractures within 1.5 cm of the fifth metatarsal distal tuberosity and have a high rate of nonunion. Fracture of the fifth metatarsal diaphysis (>1.5 cm) is associated with an increased risk of nonunion because of poor blood supply, often requiring open reduction and internal fixation. Avulsion fractures are much more common. The physical examination of the foot should always look for pain on palpation of the fifth metatarsal tuberosity. These fractures usually can be treated conservatively by immobilization in an orthopaedic boot or cast for four to six weeks (longer for diaphyseal fractures).

Lisfranc's Fracture/Sprain

This is a fracture or sprain to the base of the second metatarsal. The base of the second metatarsal is a load-bearing keystone, which locks with the

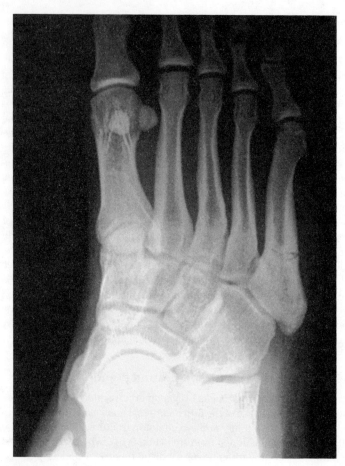

Figure 9.13 Jones fracture.

mortise of the second cuneiform bone. Causes may be direct force injuries, such as falls in a "tip-toe" position, motor-vehicle accidents, crushing injuries (e.g., run over by an automobile or stepped on by a horse), or indirect force injuries, such as other motor-vehicle accidents and windsurfing injuries. On radiographs, look for widening of the inter-metatarsal spaces and lining up with the cuneiforms. Open reduction and alignment are necessary for a good clinical outcome; surgery and stabilization/fixation of the second metatarsal keystone with either screws or Kirschner wires is a common procedure. The most feared long-term complication of this injury is significant posttraumatic arthritis.

SELECTED DISORDERS OF THE FOOT AND ANKLE

Hallux Valgus (Bunion)

The bunion (Fig. 9.14) is primarily a disorder of the first metatarsal joint in which the normal stabilizing forces, such as the plantar aponeurosis, abductor and adductor hallucis, flexor hallucis longus, and EHL, all contribute. Deviation of the proximal phalanx into valgus position and, ultimately, great toe pronation directs pressure toward the medial eminence of the metatarsal head, resulting in metatarsalgia. Women are affected more than men (10:1 ratio), presumably because of restrictive footwear, such as pointy-toed shoes. Presenting symptoms include medial eminence pain, plantar first metatarsal or lesser metatarsal head pain, and associated deformity of the medial foot. The intersection of the lines that longitudinally bisect the proximal phalanx and first metatarsal head normally is less than 15°. The hallux valgus angle is greater than 15°. Cosmetic surgery is not indicated for bunions but should be undertaken to correct a symptomatic structural deformity. Surgical correction may be considered, depending on the

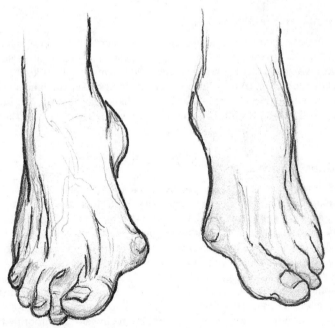

Figure 9.14 Bunion.

severity of the deformity and the associated symptoms. Surgery is discouraged in athletes and dancers, however, unless the deformity becomes debilitating, because a loss of function is almost inevitable. Proximal metatarsal osteotomies can be performed for metatarsalgia with good results, but the pain and weight-bearing center often are transferred from the first to the second to the third metatarsal head, creating similar problems.

Morton's Neuroma

This thickening of the neural tissue in a pedal digital nerve often results from trauma, previous foot surgery, compressive forces, or chronic irritation. Women are 10-fold more likely to get a neuroma of the foot. Symptoms often are pain, burning, or the sensation of "walking on a marble." Palpation of a mass or nodule in the area of pain and radiography can rule out a fracture. Treatment usually is conservative and consists of changes in footwear, nonsteroidal anti-inflammatory drugs, and corticosteroid injections. Relief is attained in approximately 80% of patients, and surgery can be offered in refractory cases.

Hammer Toe/Mallet Toe

Hammer toes most commonly involve the second toe at both joints, giving it a hammer- or claw-like appearance. Mallet toe is more subtle, involving the DIP joint of the toes and leaving a mallet-like shape. These conditions most often result from compression in tight shoes, such as high heels; other causes include diabetes, rheumatoid arthritis, and osteoarthritis. Unnatural forces shape the toes into these positions.

Sinus Tarsi Syndrome

This syndrome is characterized by pain over the lateral aspect of the ankle, and it often is misdiagnosed as a sprain. Most often, it is caused by a severe ankle inversion injury with tearing of the tarsal canal ligaments, which lie over the junction between the inferior neck of the talus, and injury to the superior aspect of the distal calcaneus (sinus tarsi). Ligaments are injured or torn, according to the severity of force, in the following order: anterior talofibular ligament, calcaneofibular ligament, cervical ligament, and interosseous talocalcaneal ligament. Diagnosis is made by pain on palpation of the sinus tarsi (palpation just below lateral malleolus), feelings of hindfoot instability, and pain that is eased by splinting the ankle in a pronated or valgus position. Radiographs usually are normal. Magnetic resonance imaging often is helpful, however, and as usual, it should be ordered to support the physical diagnosis. Treatment often is conservative, consisting of splinting and limited use of injected anesthetics and corticosteroids. Surgery involves tarsectomy and ligamentoplasty and often is effective.

Quick Look • **Foot and Ankle**

Inspect the skin. looking for gross deformity, effusion, guarding, and bruising.

Palpate the ankle, looking for focal areas of pain or effusion.

Attempt to move the foot through its ROM. If this is after a recent ankle sprain, you will need to defer some of the examination until the swelling goes down in a few days.

- **Flexion:** Ankle mortise, 50°; first MTP, 40°.
- **Extension:** Ankle mortise, 15°; first MTP, 60–75°.
- **Inversion:** Subtalar, 20°.
- **Eversion:** Subtalar, 10°.

Reflex testing if neurologic deficits, cervical stenosis, or upper motor neuron (UMN)/lower motor neuron (LMN) disorder is suspected or if the patient is preoperative or postoperative.

- **Patellar (L4), Achilles (S1):**
  - **Absent:** Neuropathy, LMN lesion.
  - **Hyperactive:** UMN lesion.

Evaluate muscles using **special tests** to isolate disorder:

- **Ankle dorsiflexion test:** To determine whether gastrocnemius or gastrocnemius–soleus is limiting motion.
  - Flex the knee joint; if you cannot dorsiflex the ankle, then the gastrocnemius is limiting.
  - Soleus should be same in either flexion or extension.
- **Anterior drawer test:** Ankle instability. Flex the patient's knee, stabilize the tibia by cupping the heel, and move the ankle mortise joint in the anteroposterior direction.
- **Flat feet test:** Observe the arch while sitting and standing.
- **Forefoot adduction test:** If the foot cannot be abducted beyond a neutral position, then correction of femoral version may be advised.

- **Homan's test:** Possible DVT (low specificity); pain (reflex) in calf with forced dorsiflexion in addition to pain on palpation.
- **Talar tilt test:** Ankle instability; inversion at the ankle causing tilting and lifting of the mortise joint.
- **Thompson test:** Achilles tendon rupture/tear. Flex the knee in a prone patient; squeezing the calf should provoke plantar flexion.
- **Tibial torsion (toeing-in) test:** An imaginary line drawn between malleoli is rotated 15° from a perpendicular line drawn from the tibial tubercle to ankle.

Order appropriate films.

- **Ankle**
  - **AP:** Good visualization of the distal tibia and fibula. No rotation between the talar dome and lateral malleolus. Follow the cortices of the tibia, fibula, and tibial plafond.
  - **Lateral:** Clear view of the AP margins of the tibia and fibula. Examine the fifth metatarsal base for an avulsion fracture. The talar dome is a smooth arc.
  - **Mortise:** Ankle mortise joint. Consider a hot light to inspect for bone fragments. No widening of uniform joint space. Intact medial clear space (<4 mm). Inspect talar dome. Lateral tibiofibular clear space <5.5 mm.
- **Foot**
  - **AP:** View the first and second MTP. Check alignment of the navicular bone with talus. Check midtarsal joints for fracture. Check alignment of the second metatarsal with the second cuneiform. Scan the phalanges and metatarsals. All other bone cortices are smooth and intact.
  - **Lateral:** View back to front, and check the talus, calcaneus, talar body and neck, metatarsal alignment, and fifth metatarsal base. Inspect the talar dome, subtalar joint, and talar neck. Evaluate the calcaneus for fracture. Calculate the Bohler's angle (<20°). Examine the base of the fifth metatarsal avulsion fracture.
  - **Internal oblique:** Scan the film back to front, and identify all of the bones of the foot. Check the anterior talus. Examine the calcaneus for fracture/avulsion fragments. Check the intertarsals and tarsometatarsals. Check the metatarsals and phalanges for fracture. The fourth metatarsal should align with the medial cortex of the cuboid.

SELECTED REFERENCES

AAOS. Morton's neuroma. Available at: http://orthoinfo.aaos.org/fact/thr_report.cfm?Thread_ID=233&topcategory=Foot. Accessed December 26, 2006.

Alvarez R, Haddad RJ, Gould N, Trevino S. The simple bunion: anatomy at the first metatarsophalangeal joint of the great toe. Foot Ankle 1984;4:229.

Andrish JT. Meniscal injuries in children and adolescents J Am Acad Orthop Surg 1996;4:231–237.

Coughlin MJ. Hallux valgus. J Bone Joint Surg Am 1996;78:932–966.

Gosele A, Schulenburg J, Ochsner PE. Early functional treatment of a fifth metatarsal fracture using an orthopedic boot. Swiss Surg 1997;3(2):81–84.

Klausner VB, McKeigue ME. The sinus tarsi syndrome: a cause of chronic ankle pain. Available at: http://physsportsmed.com/issues/2000/05-00/Klausner.htm. Accessed April 12, 2006.

Larson RL, Taillon M. Anterior cruciate ligament insufficiency: principles of treatment. J Am Acad Orthop Surg 1994;2:26–35.

Mayo Clinic Staff. Hammer toe and mallet toe. Available at: http://www.mayoclinic.com/invoke.cfm?id=DS00480. Accessed April 15, 2006.

Mulier T, Reynders P, Dereymaeker G, Broos P. Severe Lisfrancs injuries: primary arthrodesis or ORIF? Foot Ankle Int 2002;23:902–905.

Patel R, Haddad F. Metatarsal fractures: break it like Beckham. Available at: http://www.sportsinjurybulletin.com/archive/metatarsal-fractures.html. Accessed March 20, 2006.

Rockwood CA, Green DP, Bucholz RW, eds. Rockwood and Green's Fractures in Adults, Vol. 2. 3rd Ed. Philadelphia: Lippincott, 1991:2155–2156.

Steinberg GG, Akins CM, Baran DT. Orthopaedics in Primary Care. 3rd Ed. Baltimore: Lippincott Williams and Wilkins, 1999:287–288.

Osteoporosis tests. Available at: http://orthoinfo.aaos.org/fact/thr_report.cfm?thread_id=176&topcategory=Osteoporosis. Accessed January 22, 2006.

Index